Occupational Therapy:
New Perspectives

Occupational Therapy: New Perspectives

Edited by

JENNIFER CREEK

Course Leader, Occupational Therapy, University of Teesside

Consulting Editor in Occupational Therapy

CLEPHANE HUME

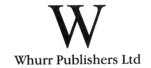

Whurr Publishers Ltd

© 1998 Whurr Publishers Ltd
First published 1998 by
Whurr Publishers Ltd
19b Compton Terrace, London N1 2UN, England

Reprinted 2000 and 2002

British Library Cataloguing in Publication Data
A catalogue record for this book is available from
the British Library.

ISBN 1 86156 088 5

Printed and bound in the UK by Athenaeum Press Ltd,
Gateshead, Tyne & Wear

Contents

Preface

The profession of occupational therapy emerged in the early part of the twentieth century, founded by a number of people with a humane interest in the condition of patients in long-stay psychiatric institutions. The first occupational therapists were trained in the use of arts and crafts, and their job was to structure the day of hospital residents into a stimulating pattern of work, rest and play. They worked under the supervision of doctors; the doctor provided the direction and the occupational therapist carried out programmes of activity.

In the past eight decades, occupational therapists have developed from the handmaidens of the medical profession into semi-autonomous, largely self-regulating professionals, working in many different fields of practice in an increasing number of countries throughout the world. Underpinning this rapid expansion is a concomitant growth in practical, clinical skills and in the theoretical base of the profession. Beginning in the 1950s, occupational therapists began to use and adapt theories borrowed from other disciplines, such as medicine and psychology, to explain and extend their practice. As the profession matured, it started to develop its own theories and principles, based on an awareness of the human need for a balanced but changing range of activities throughout life to support health and wellbeing.

The idea of editing a collection of critical essays on current concepts of occupational therapy came to me gradually as I listened to papers at conferences, read professional journals and talked to colleagues. There is a renewed sense of excitement and discovery within the profession but we still lack a forum where people can describe their work more fully and, perhaps, stimulate academic debate. We are not yet confident enough to be self-critical, we are at the stage of being pleased with ourselves because we understand theory building, yet there is a need for energetic discussion and argument to take our ideas forward.

Having thought about these issues for a year or two, I decided to find out if occupational therapists could be persuaded to expose their work in progress to the critical gaze of colleagues. At a national conference, I approached some of the people whose work I most admire and asked if they would like to contribute to a collection of papers on current issues in occupational therapy. The response was universally positive. My initial idea was to make a collection of British writings as a snapshot of how British occupational therapists are developing in the 1990s. However, exciting work is emerging all over the world and I could not resist including papers from Hong Kong and Australia. In the end, the difficulty was to limit the number of contributions because so much recent work demands attention.

The first chapter sets the scene by exploring the relationship between occupation and health. Occupational therapists have, for nearly a century, expressed belief in a relationship between what people do and their health, yet we are still in the early stages of finding an explanation for that relationship. This chapter makes a substantial contribution to the process.

The next two chapters examine in depth two concepts that are central to the practice of occupational therapy. Chapter 2 reviews what has been written about the nature of purposeful activity and considers why this remains an important tool in the occupational therapist's repertoire. Chapter 3 describes a theory to explain the value of person-centred practice and demonstrates how this approach, characteristic of occupational therapy intervention, fits in with wider health care systems and policies.

Chapters 4 to 7 focus on different aspects of the occupational therapy process which have been recognised in recent years as essential components of practice. Chapter 4 looks at various models of clinical reasoning and considers some influences on how occupational therapists reason. Chapter 5 reviews our current understanding of reflection and addresses how it can help us to improve our clinical practice. Chapter 6 is a provocative account of the difficulties occupational therapists might have in living up to the high moral ideals they claim to espouse. Chapter 7 takes a proactive approach to the problem of finding a realistic measure of the outcomes of occupational therapy intervention.

The penultimate chapter explores occupational therapists' anxieties about their role and function through consideration of the ways in which they try to communicate with others. The issue of professional identity is linked with use of language.

The last chapter is the only one not written by an occupational therapist. It offers an outsider's vision of the tension experienced by the therapist between wanting to work with the client, from his or her perspective, and needing to demonstrate professional effectiveness to managers and others.

These essays do not constitute a definitive account of the current state of thinking in occupational therapy. They are intended to stimulate interest in academic debate and to provoke a critical response. Read and enjoy them!

Contributors

Rosemary Barnitt PhD DipCOT
Rosemary Barnitt completed her doctoral studies in 1996 on the topic of ethics in health care. She is reader in occupational therapy at the University of Southampton.

Jennifer Creek Dip COT
Jennifer Creek qualified as an occupational therapist and an art therapist. She has worked in the fields of adult mental health, learning disabilities and occupational therapy education.

Mary Jenkins DipCOT, BSc, DPhil
Mary Jenkins is a part-time lecturer at the University of Ulster and Belfast Institute of Further and Higher Education and a full-time community practitioner.

Mary Perks
Mary Perks is an artist and art therapist, trained in France and at St Albans and specialising in mental health. She is also a counsellor, supervisor and workshop and retreat leader.

Susan Ryan
Susan Ryan is a reader in educational development in health sciences at the University of East London. Her doctoral study looks at how newly qualified occupational therapists have made meaning from their educational experiences.

Kit Sinclair MSC, BSOT, OTR
Kit Sinclair, assistant professor in occupational therapy at the Hong Kong Polytechnic University is presently pursuing her PhD on the subject of reflective practice. Trained in the United States, she has worked as a clinician and educator in Asia for over 30 years.

Penny Spreadbury
Penny Spreadbury is working on a rehabilitation unit for people with neurological conditions. Previously, she spent three years developing an outcome measure for occupational therapists.

Ann Wilcock DipCOT(UK), BAppScOT, GradDipPublic Health, PhD
Ann Wilcock joined the University of South Australia after 15 years of clinical practice. She was founding editor of *Occupational Science: Australia*.

Chapter 1
A theory of occupation and health

ANN WILCOCK

Introduction

In this chapter a theory about the relationship between occupation and health will be presented. The theory, which suggests that engagement in occupation is a central, evolutionary mechanism for the maintenance and promotion of health, was researched and developed using a 'history of ideas' approach. Should future practice be based on it, such a theory would enable occupational therapists to make a distinctive and substantial contribution to improving the health and wellbeing of both communities and individuals.

The theory was prompted by the directions of the 'new' public health movement and the World Health Organisation's (WHO) calls for all health professionals to reorient their practice towards primary health care, the prevention of illness, disease and disability and the promotion of health and wellbeing (World Health Organisation 1978, 1986). In these directives it was recognised that health is multifactorial and that many different strategies, initiatives and orientations would improve the experience of health globally. Such recognition provided the impetus to question what could be the particular and distinctive role of occupational therapists in a reoriented practice.

Occupational therapists have long held that there is a link between engagement in occupation and positive health. Although recent practice has concentrated on illness models and adaptation to handicap, a resurgence of concern about occupation as an holistic concept has occurred, as evidenced by interest in the 'Model of Human Occupation' (Kielhofner 1980a, Kielhofner and Burke 1980; 1980b; Kielhofner, Burke Igi and 1980) and the emerging discipline of occupational science (Kielhofner 1985; Yerxa, Clark, Frank et al. 1989). Despite this interest, the idea of a relationship between occupation and health has not been researched in any depth. Intuitively, it appears to have value but until recently occupational therapists have not sought to establish, or base practice upon, a theory about health that is unique to the profession.

The first steps to providing a direction for reorienting future practice appeared to be threefold: an increased understanding of human occupation; an increased understanding of ideas about health, and the development of a theory about the relationship between health and occupation, from an occupational perspective. The ultimate aim was towards a theory, as distinct from a model of practice or frame of reference, which could be distinctive to occupational therapists enabling them to make unique, varied, recognisable and satisfying contributions to global and individual health. A history-of-ideas approach was deemed the most appropriate for such research.

It is important to consider the rationale for using this methodology. Because of the complexity of factors associated with the health of people engaging in occupation in ever changing environments, the restrictions imposed by so-called 'scientific' methods of analysis are not appropriate for developing theory. Indeed, in recent years, many qualitative approaches, such as grounded theory, have been recognised as more effective tools (Glaser and Strauss 1967).

History-of-ideas method

A history-of-ideas approach, which is grounded in the context of ideas from many disciplines, offers similar advantages to grounded theory. It brings together and analyses, from new and different perspectives, notions, philosophies and theories that have been widely accepted as reasonable interpretations of complex issues. It recognises that many minds have reflected on important questions relating to the human condition over thousands of years, and that reviewing the results of such deliberations from a new perspective may provide unexpected answers that have potential value for people today. The term 'history of ideas' was introduced by Arthur Lovejoy in the 1920s for the study of ideas that 'disregard national and linguistic boundary lines', are widely diffused and cross barriers between disciplines (Lovejoy 1936, p. 182).

The human phenomenon of engagement in occupation is certainly one which disregards boundaries, and has been considered from many angles according to the interests of different disciplines. It is an appropriate issue for theory development, as Lovejoy proposed that the task of a history of ideas is to assist with 'interpretation and unification' when theorists or researchers seek to correlate things which may appear unconnected; in this case, the correlation sought is between health and occupation.

Histories of ideas use critical text analysis, centring on concepts and how changes in their meaning and associations alter according to context, so the research led to a voyage of discovery from health promotion and public health through to evolution, anthropology, sociology, philosophy, ethology, socio-biology, genetics, labour studies, psychology, ecology and Neural Darwinism as well as occupational therapy. During the research and development stage of the theory the evolutionary, biological and sociocultural contexts and sources of ideas were considered and clarified, and their similarities and differences analysed. Following this step, theoretical reflection in relation to developing a particular view of health and occupation could begin. Outlining the direction of the study was a dynamic and changing process as unexpected issues emerged and previously discarded ideas became relevant as fresh connections were made. From the foundation laid by immersion in the literature, by open-minded reflection and by the process of writing itself, a critical viewpoint was facilitated and a theory emerged.

The theory

It is important to ask what makes a good theory. According to Stephen Hawking a good theory, which meets the criterion of current empirical accuracy, must be based upon few arbitrary elements derived from multiple and ongoing observations and it must have predictive capacity (Hawking 1988, p. 10). The theory outlined here is based upon only two arbitrary elements: first that humans are occupational beings and, second, that engagement in occupation is a major evolutionary mechanism for health. It is derived from multiple and ongoing observations of people engaging in occupations across cultures and time. The theory definitely predicts that people will continue to engage in occupations and that this will impact upon their health, although the form of the occupations will change according to sociocultural evolution. In line with criteria set forth by Stevenson in *Seven Theories of Human Nature*, the theory also provides 'a background theory of the nature of the world' which is compatible with this view of the occupational nature of people, 'a diagnosis of what is wrong' in terms of health from this view, along with 'a prescription for putting it right' (Stevenson 1987, p. 9).

The evolutionary context of the theory, in line with current scientific thought, accepts that living matter evolved naturally from non-living matter (Stavrianos 1988). Charles Darwin's theory of evolution by natural selection demonstrates a way in which 'simplicity could change into complexity' (Dawkins 1976, p. 39). His theory is based on the empirical observations that, despite a tendency for parental traits to be passed to their offspring, there are considerable and noticeable variations between individuals, and that within species more are born than can survive, requiring a struggle for existence. This leads to those with 'certain inherited variants' having an increased chance of 'surviving and reproducing', and results in the accumulation of favoured variants that will, over extended periods, produce new forms of life (Jones 1992, p. 9). Gregor Mendel's experiments with plant species provided the answer to the 'causes of the variations on which natural selection acts' (Campbell 1988, p. 67) and, in recent times, 'the discovery of the structure and function of DNA has made clear the nature of the hereditary variations upon which natural selection operates' (Dyson 1979, p. 49). Genetic recombination, which theoretically can 'create nearly an infinite number of different organisms simply by reshuffling the immense amount of genetic differences between the DNA of any two parents', means that there is considerable variation between individuals (McHenry 1989, p. 280). Indeed, diversity and individual uniqueness is the consistent message of evolutionary studies (Jones 1992, p. 9). Individual uniqueness, particularly in relation to biological characteristics and capacities, influences engagement in occupation, as well as individual health outcomes, as a result of occupational behaviours.

Having briefly clarified the context, two key issues associated with the theory will be discussed in the next section of the chapter. The first issue concerns what is meant when occupational therapists and occupational scientists talk about 'humans as occupational beings' and the second the concept of occupation as an evolutionary mechanism for health.

Humans as occupational beings

This is a powerful description that requires careful consideration and poses many questions about the nature of occupation, its evolution and its purposes. All animals engage in occupations. For example, most hunt and forage for food, care for their young and engage in social rituals. Some, such as chimpanzees, use tools for such tasks, and most people will have observed how dogs, cats and budgerigars learn to play with or without objects. Occupational behaviour differs according to species characteristics and to each species' range of capacities. Archeological and anthropological opinion suggests that, throughout the existence of our species, humans and earlier hominids, engaged in occupation in a more complex manner than other animals. Indeed, complex occupational behaviour is said by some to differentiate humans from the other species (Bronowski 1973; Leakey 1981). It has allowed us to change, or adapt to and survive healthily, in many different environments.

Some capacities and characteristics of the human species that appear to make considerable contributions to complex occupational behaviour have been identified. Upright walking, hand dexterity, stereoscopic vision, language and social nature are prime examples that Campbell suggests have 'overwhelming significance' and when 'added together separate all humans from all other animals' (Campbell 1988, p. 47). In evolutionary terms 'the shape of cells, tissues, organs, and finally the whole animal – is the largest single basis for behaviour' (Edelman 1992, p. 49). The central nervous system is particularly important because it is the brain that co-ordinates and controls engagement in occupation.

It is in the cerebral cortex that the processes occur that make humans most different from other animals, such as their capacity to analyse, organise, understand, produce, judge, plan, activate, formulate and execute complex occupation (Kolb and Whishaw 1990, Ornstein and Sobel 1988). Such cortical functions give humans the 'capacity to adapt culturally . . . to insulate themselves from the environment and to exploit the environment' (Campbell 1988, p. 55).

Although the range of human capacities is, on the whole, common to the species, individual variation is the rule. This results in every person having a range of occupational capacities and needs that is distinct to him or her; as Ornstein and Sobel (1988, p. 57) contend talents 'are not given equally to all of us'. The genetic difference is increased by the human capacity to learn from the environment. Human young are born early in the process of developing abilities and independence skills, so they have a long period of immaturity when they are exposed and extremely susceptible to learning from their social situation. This early period of socialisation allows infants to learn, by absorption, about how to survive in their particular environment. Each environment, however, differs according to ecological, cultural, social and familial factors, as well as the timing of events and occupational opportunities, increasing further the uniqueness and development of each individual.

Occupational behaviour, then, is a result of the processes of natural selection throughout evolution as organisms have adapted to their environment, of genetic inheritance, of individual biological structure and form, of ontogenesis, of sociocultural and familial factors and of opportunity, experience and learning.

Over the past 2–3 million years, human occupation has become extremely complex because of continual evolution, the development of occupational technology and the social structures and values that accompany it. Occupation, despite modern usage of the term, is much more than paid employment. It is a central aspect of the human experience because it encompasses all the things that people do, whether work, play or rest, obligatory or chosen, physical, mental or social, biological or sociocultural in origin. That people 'do' is so much a part of the ordinary fabric of life that it is taken for granted. Although people engage in different occupations according to their culture, society and its values, and experience, the meaning of occupations differs for each individual, and it seems important to bring to the forefront of our thinking that all people feel a need to engage in occupations that have meaning for them and that use their particular interests and capacities.

Such ideas suggest that occupation is an innate behaviour; that it is an integral aspect of humanness; that it may even define humanness; that doing and being have an intimate relationship and that occupation has biological as well as social functions. Humans can be described as occupational beings because of this.

Occupation as an evolutionary mechanism for health

The second issue to be considered is the claim that engagement in occupation is a major evolutionary mechanism for health. Most people in post-industrial societies consider health from the perspective of medical science, which is attuned to the task of restoring health following illness or of preventing illness occurring. In contrast to this view, an understanding of health as a natural phenomenon was sought by examining the possible underlying relationship between health and occupation. The subsequent exploration of ideas about the biological bases and evolution of occupation, from the first known hominids through to the present time, has led to the proposal that the evolutionary functions of occupation for all animals are survival and health.

Survival is recognised as the primary drive of humans, as of all other animals (Lorenz 1983). Survival of individual humans is the outcome of occupations that provide for the essential needs of the organism: food, water, temperature control and supportive social, ecological and material environments. Health is the outcome of each organism having all essential sustenance and safety needs met and of having physical, mental and social capacities maintained, exercised and in balance. This is achieved through occupation; through what people do day by day. Engagement in occupation depends, in turn, on a level of health able to provide the energy, drive and functional attributes necessary for such engagement. Additionally, the healthy survival of the species depends on humans' capacity to live in harmony within an environment that can continue to provide basic requirements; to ensure the continued acquisition of these requirements and to provide health, safety and education for the next generation (Wilcock 1998).

This theory is complementary to a widely held view that the principal goal of evolution is genomic reproduction. Positive health enhances survival and reproductive success because, at the very least, as reproduction only occurs during a particular stage of the life cycle, to reach this stage individuals have to resist disease and death. Engagement in occupation is not only required for survival to the point of reproduction but also for a long time after to provide the wherewithal for the immature of the species because human young have lengthy childhoods. 'Kin selection', which extends the concept of Darwinian 'fitness' to include individuals who share genes (Campbell 1988), accounts, at least in part, for altruistic behaviours and occupations that support biological parents in this task.

It is probably fair to suggest that this concept of health has received little attention. This may be, partly, because natural survival and health-maintaining functions are built into the organism to just go on working so, unless asked to consider such factors, people do not give much conscious thought to them. Additionally, the basic functions of occupation are now obscured, particularly in post-industrial societies, by the social functions and value given to occupation. But, looking backwards, it can be claimed that, for more than two million years, hominids and humans flourished, despite a shorter lifespan than at present, along with other animals in a natural environment without the advantages of modern medicine. Many anthropologists, ecologists, philosophers, physicians and others assert that humans in a state of nature have an instinct for health that modern humans have lost (Virey 1828). This assertion is supported by reports of some explorers following their initial contacts with people of primitive cultures. Captain James Cook provided one example when he recorded in his journal (1768–71), that the natives of the Pacific islands he visited were 'happy, healthy and full of vigour' (Wharton 1893, p. 323). Such reports pose the question of why this might be.

One answer, which fits well with this theory, is provided by Ornstein and Sobel's (1988, pp. 11–12) proposal that 'the major role of the brain is to mind the body and maintain health', because the brain, by making 'countless adjustments', continually maintains stability between our 'social worlds, our mental and emotional lives, and our internal physiology'. They provide substantial physiological evidence and medical research that supports their view. In this theory it is suggested that occupational 'needs', which recognise the human organism as a whole in interaction with the environment, have an integral role in the central nervous system process of maintaining stability and health and promoting wellbeing (Wilcock 1993).

Occupational needs warn when a problem occurs in order to protect and prevent potential disorder. They do this by prompting action in an 'integrated response to the self system', with a main goal to 'ensure its own survival' (Csiksentmihalyi 1990). This type of need aims at immediate effects to satisfy or alleviate discomfort, such as hunger, cold, fear, boredom, tension, anxiety, pain, fatigue, anger or loneliness. Occupation undertaken in response to such need, although effective in the short term, may or may not be health promoting in the long term. Loneliness may, for example, lead to substance abuse to mask the unpleasant experience. In such a case it is likely to be the social and occupational milieux that encourage a particular response pattern.

Occupational needs also prompt use of capacities so that the organism will flourish and reach potential. This type of need is experienced in a positive sense, such as a need to be creative, expend energy, explore, walk, talk, use ideas, express thoughts, listen or look, spend time alone or with others and so on. Such needs prevent disorder by activating use of capacities, balancing overuse or underuse. If capacities are over or under used people feel fatigue, stress and boredom or burnout, which can lead to decreased immunity to illness and increased susceptibility to accidents. 'We become adapted to the lack of use of our organic and mental systems by degenerating . . . In order to reach his optimum state, the human being must actualize all his potentialities' (Carrel 1935, p.178-179). Humans' occupational needs go beyond the instinctive survival behaviours of many other animals, so the meeting of such needs is central to 'how nature intended human beings to live' (Coon 1972, p.393) and to live healthily.

The need for purpose, satisfaction, fulfilment and pleasure is also integral to the occupational nature of humans and their healthy survival. These needs reward and provide feedback to the organism that encourages further use of capacities towards potential. Occupation 'determines the chief rhythm of our life, balances it, and gives meaning and significance. An organ that does not work atrophies and the mind that does not work becomes dumb' (Sigerist 1955, pp.254–5).

To test this notion about occupational needs, a questionnaire was administered to 150 subjects, with ages ranging from 6 to 98 years. The majority reported that the satisfactory meeting of these of needs affects their mental, physical and social health in a positive way. Ninety-nine percent admitted they had experienced discomfort that prompted action, and almost all of these had responded to the prompt in some way to alleviate the discomfort; 99 percent also admitted to experiencing a need to use their capacities and to have experienced a need for purpose, satisfaction, fulfilment or pleasure. Over 95 percent agreed that they had responded to both types of needs. If they did not respond, most reported experiencing discomfort of the type described above (Wilcock, Dean and Sturgul 1993).

Society, occupation and health

It is not an accident that the occupational nature of humans has focused energies towards developing societies to meet such needs. Meeting them facilitates wellbeing because the health-maintaining-and-promoting ingredients of occupations are related to people's individual capacities and purposes. They can promote homeostasis by balancing social, physical, mental and rest activity; can be satisfying and challenging; can enable growth and development towards self-actualisation, and are especially effective if they are largely self-chosen, socially valued and rewarded. Other important factors integral to the individual experience of a health-promoting occupation include the fact that it is undertaken in an occupationally just society and in an environment that is safe, supportive and unpolluted. It is also evident that communities have the same occupational requirements for their wellbeing as individuals.

The World Health Organisation (WHO) has recognised a close relationship between health and wellbeing. In fact, in its definition of health, maintained since 1946, the WHO describes it as physical, mental

and social wellbeing and not just the absence of illness. In the Ottawa
Charter for Health Promotion (World Health Organisation 1986), international health authorities also recognise the benefits of occupation to
health and wellbeing. In this document it is stated that:

> to reach a state of complete physical, mental and social wellbeing, an
> individual or group must be able to identify and to realize aspira-
> tions, to satisfy needs, and to change or cope with the environment.

Health, the document goes on, 'cannot be separated from other goals'
because it 'is created and lived by people within the settings of their
everyday life; where they learn, work, play and love'.

To explore the relationship between occupation and wellbeing a
survey of seven convenience cluster samples, selected from high school
students, an elderly citizens' village, family units, a suburban neighbour-
hood, a city shopping centre, churchgoers and fourth-year occupational
therapy students, was undertaken. One hundred and thirty eight
subjects were asked with what situation or environment they associated
a feeling of wellbeing and, of these, 60 percent of the responses were
definitely related to occupation. They included answers categorised as
work, leisure, rest, religious practices, selfless activity, self-care and
achievement. This total does not take into account any occupations
associated with social relationships, which was the single most frequent
response (56.5 percent), or spiritual (as opposed to religious) practices
that could have added a further 8.7 percent. These figures total more
than 100 percent because people could give more than one response
(Wilcock et al. 1991).

Psychologists of the 'Hormic school' recognised that 'primitive
instinctive energy can be directed from its natural goal towards alternative ends that are [perceived to be] of a greater value' (Knight and Knight
1957, p. 177). The materialism of the present day is a prime example.
Although notions about instinct and drive are out of fashion within
current psychological theory, there appears to be some value in considering how the process of redirection enables individuals to make
occupational choices according to the particular circumstances in which
they find themselves. Indeed, it is on this process of redirection and
choice that 'all the highest achievements of humanity' depend (Knight
and Knight 1957, p. 177).

Social barriers to healthy occupational choice

The downside to the mechanism of choice is that it allows people to act
'against the millennial wisdom that natural selection had built into the
biological fabric of the species' (Csikszenmihalyi and Csikszenmihalyi
1988, pp. 20–1). Their capacity to ignore biological occupational needs

means that people may make choices with detrimental health consequences. In the present day it is difficult to make healthy choices because the gradual evolution of complex occupational structures in response to cultural forces has become a hindrance in teasing out the survival and health-maintaining behaviours that once dominated occupational engagement.

Medical science has developed as much to overcome the problems and diseases caused by our changed occupational lifestyles as it has to address the problems of genetic or infectious diseases. The diseases caused by lifestyle, which create most concern in affluent societies, include cardiovascular, respiratory, nutritional, mental and sexually transmitted disorders, cancer and accidents. Their major causes, identified to date, include cigarette smoking, alcohol and drug abuse, poor eating habits, unsafe sex, decreased levels of exercise and fitness and stress (Last 1987). All these causes can be related to occupational issues. For example, coronary heart disease (French and Caplan 1972), disorders of the digestive and immune systems (McQuade and Aikman 1974), as well as depressive illness can result from 'all day-every day' stressors such as occupational imbalance, deprivation or alienation. Yet these are rarely the focus of medical intervention or even an issue of concern.

Occupational imbalance occurs when people engage in too much of the same type of activity, limiting the use of their various capacities; occupational deprivation when factors beyond them limit an individual's choice or opportunity, and occupational alienation occurs when people are unable to meet basic occupational needs or use their particular capacities because of sociocultural factors. All have undoubtedly increased with the evolved complexity of human lifestyles, cultural values, societal rules, sophisticated technology and subsequent ecological detachment. Stress-related illness as a result of occupational alienation, deprivation and imbalance has also increased, and is more pronounced and prevalent in 'atomistic societies', than in 'organic communities' in which natural functions, role perspectives, mutual interdependence and intrinsic relations are stressed (Mijuskovic 1992).

Let us consider briefly, for example, how corporate and government initiatives across major post-industrial nations have resulted in many people in paid employment now being expected to take on increased duties and to spend longer hours on work tasks without extra rewards, afraid to refuse because of decreasing job opportunities. Health breakdowns caused by this are increasing (Gare 1995; Schor 1991). At the other end of the paid employment continuum, physical and mental ill-health is also on the increase, having often been found to accompany the experiences of the unemployed because, in large part, of a lack of opportunity to engage in satisfying and socially valued occupation (Jahoda 1988; Smith 1987; Winefield and Tiggerman 1991).

Prolonged occupational imbalance, deprivation or alienation can be considered risk factors in their own right, or lead to the development of health risk behaviours such as smoking or substance abuse. They may also occur as a result of other occupational risk factors such as workaholism, division of labour or occupational inequities at a societal level. All can lead to pre-clinical health disorders such as boredom, burnout, decreased fitness, brain or liver dysfunction and changes in blood pressure, body weight, emotional state and sleep patterns, and ultimately to disease, disability or death.

There are many underlying factors to this unhealthy scenario. They too can be described as occupational at a national or community level. The type of economy, national priorities and policies and cultural values that create occupational institutions and activities at a societal level can lead to risk factors such as overcrowding, loneliness, substance abuse, lack of opportunity to develop potential, imbalance between diet and activity and ecological breakdown. The type of economy, such as whether it is nomadic, agricultural, industrial, post-industrial, capitalist or socialist, for example, will determine the amount and type of technology in daily living, employment opportunities and how long and in what circumstances people carry out obligatory or chosen occupations. National policies and priorities, such as policies towards economic growth or sustainable ecology, the wealth and power of multi-national organisations or self-generating community development have a direct effect upon the day-by-day occupations of individuals, on the legislative and fiscal institutions that provide rules by which people live, and on commercial and material activities and management of the environment. Such policies will both drive and be influenced by dominant cultural values, including such ideas as the work ethic, occupational justice and equity between class, age, gender and ability, local regulations, social services and directions for the education of the young (Wilcock 1998). Blaxter's findings from a survey undertaken in the United Kingdom with a sample of 9000 adults support this view in that 'not only socio-economic circumstances and the external environment, but also the individual's psycho-social environment – carry rather more weight, as determinants of health, than healthy or unhealthy behaviours' (Blaxter 1990, p. 233).

It is possible, therefore, for these same underlying factors to be facilitatory to the experience of positive health and wellbeing for both communities and individuals. This is only if they provide equitable opportunities for people to develop potential, creativity and balanced use of capacities, to experience satisfaction, meaning and purpose, stability and support, belonging and sharing and being able to contribute in a way that is socially valued yet maintains natural resources.

If the underlying occupational determinants are favourable, the results should be apparent in what can be termed 'occupational indicators of health status'. Individual indicators include energy and alertness, a range of activities, flexibility, interest, contentment, commitment, the ability to relax and sleep, time for others and openness to new challenges. These are likely to be compatible with more conventional health status indicators such as appropriate height/weight ratios, normal blood pressures, cholesterol levels and lung function (Wilcock 1998). Health and wellbeing result from being in tune with our occupational nature.

Conclusion

Having outlined the main concepts of this theory about occupation and health, it is possible to suggest, albeit briefly, a diagnosis of what is wrong from the particular perspective of the theory and to suggest possible corrective action. In contrast to the occupational behaviour of early humans, which was in harmony and balance with 'natural' health, at present it is out of step, being 'born from the whims of scientific discoveries, from the appetites of men, their illusions, their theories, and their desires' but 'without any knowledge of our real nature' (Carrel 1935, p. 14). To demonstrate such knowledge, any comprehensive theory of human nature should include the all-embracing phenomenon of occupational behaviour, but few do. Karl Marx's view that labour is our species' nature, and that the further it evolves from the natural the more alienating and unhealthy it becomes, comes close, but even this became watered down by sociopolitical rhetoric (Marx 1844).

Why is it that human occupation has been so little considered? Perhaps because the need 'to do' is so natural, so much a part of being, that humans have failed to recognise it as an entity. Instead, they have reduced the holistic concept of occupation by dividing it and then made it more complex by endowing specific aspects with particular values. Additionally, people's ongoing need for purpose, challenge, new and different pursuits and for exploring ways of making their lives easier has led to a situation in which the products and results of human occupation have assumed more importance than 'natural' human need.

In healthcare, although it has been recognised by world and public health authorities that occupational behaviours can lead to positive or negative health outcomes, there is little action at this level to promote the positive or inhibit the negative. It is left then for health workers with a particular interest in occupation, such as occupational therapists, to promulgate the concept and take action.

Occupational therapy, a profession with particular strengths in conceptualising humans from an occupational perspective, has a unique but repressed history. Dominated by medical science since its very early days, this largely female profession has not been encouraged, until recently, to consider its unique contribution in terms of theory. Instead, occupational therapists have considered whatever aspects of 'divided occupation' are in vogue according to medical directives and the theories of other disciplines, from the creative through to self care and paid employment. Insight into this situation provides opportunity for corrective action. It is possible, particularly if occupational therapists seriously pursue the study of humans as occupational beings and apply their findings to public as well as conventional health scenarios, that the lack of insight into occupational needs and their effect on health can be addressed at last.

The study of health, from this perspective, requires serious and immediate consideration, research and action at individual, community and environmental levels. Addressing the lack of awareness of our occupational natures has the potential to influence social, political, economic and health policies so that they are more in tune with our occupational natures, self-sustaining 'natural' health and ecological balance. More concrete solutions do not seem advisable as theories of human nature that are prescriptive, such as Marxist communism, do not allow sufficient flexibility to allow solutions to be responsive to contextual and evolutionary change.

What can be done to combat the occupational inequities that may mean less-than-optimal health and wellbeing in the future? Recognition, debate and open discussion of how occupational opportunities for people differ from community to community is required. Exploration of the underlying reasons for these differences and how they impact on health and wellbeing needs to be undertaken within and by each community. This is one of the best approaches to increase awareness and promote action about causes and effects of occupational alienation, deprivation and imbalance. It also has the potential to provide support and encouragement for self-reliant, self-chosen occupation that gives meaning, purpose and social approval.

References

Blaxter M (1990) Health and Lifestyles. London and New York: Tavistock/Routledge.
Bronowski J (1973) The Ascent of Man. London: British Broadcasting Corporation.
Campbell BG (1988) Humankind Emerging. 5 edn. New York: HarperCollins.
Carrel A (1935) Man, the Unknown. London: Burns & Oates.
Coon CS (1972) The Hunting Peoples. London: Jonathan Cape.
Csikszentmihalyi M (1990) Flow: the Psychology of Optimal Experience. New York: Harper Perennial.
Csikszentmihalyi M, Csikszentmihalyi IS (eds) (1988) Optimal Experience: Psychological Studies of Flow in Consciousness. Cambridge: Cambridge University Press.
Dawkins R (1976) The Selfish Gene. Oxford: Oxford University Press.
Dyson F (1979) The argument from design. In Dixon B (ed.) (1989) From Creation to Chaos: Classic Writings in Science. Oxford: Basil Blackwell.

Edelman G (1992) Bright Air, Brilliant Fire: On the Matter of the Mind. London: Penguin.

French JRP, Caplan RD (1972) Organizational Stress and Individual Strain. In Marrow AJ (ed). The Failure of Success. New York: Amacon.

Gare S (1995) The age of overwork. The Weekend Australian Review (April 8–9): 2–3.

Glaser B, Strauss A (1967) The Discovery of Grounded Theory: Strategies for Qualitative Research. New York: Aldine.

Hawking SW (1988) A Brief History of Time. Toronto: Bantam Books.

Jahoda M (1988) Economic recession and mental health: some conceptual issues. Journal of Social Issues 44(4): 13–23.

Jones S (1992) The nature of evolution. In Jones S, Martin R, Pilbeam D (eds). The Cambridge Encyclopedia of Human Evolution. Cambridge: Cambridge University Press.

Kielhofner G (1980a) A model of human occupation, part 2. Ontogenesis from the perspective of human adaptation. American Journal of Occupational Therapy 34(10): 657–63.

Kielhofner G (1980b) A model of human occupation, part 3. Benign and vicious cycles. American Journal of Occupational Therapy 34(11): 731–7.

Kielhofner G (1985) Model of Human Occupation, Theory and Application. Philadelphia PA: FA Davis.

Kielhofner G, Burke JP (1980) A model of human occupation, Part 1. Conceptual framework and content. American Journal of Occupational Therapy 34(9): 572–81.

Kielhofner G, Burke JP, Igi CH (1980) A model of human occupation, Part 4. Assessment and intervention. American Journal of Occupational Therapy 34(12): 777–88.

Last JM (1987) Public Health and Human Ecology. East Norwalk CT: Appleton & Lange.

Leakey R (1981) The Making of Mankind. London: Michael Joseph.

Lorenz K (1983/1987) The Waning of Humaneness. Boston MA: Little Brown.

Lovejoy AO (1936) The study of the history of ideas. In King P (ed.) (1983) The History of Ideas. London and Canberra: Croom Helm.

Marx K (1844/1992) Economic and philosophical manuscripts. In Livingstone R, Benton G (translators) Karl Marx: Early Writings. London: Penguin Classics.

McHenry HM (1989) Evolution. In Kuyper A, Kuyper J (eds) The Social Science Encyclopedia. Revised edn. London and New York: Routledge & Kegan Paul.

McQuade W, Aikman A (1974) Stress. New York: Dutton.

Mijuskovic B (1992) Organic communities, atomistic societies, and loneliness. Journal of Sociology and Social Welfare 19(2): 147–64.

Ornstein R, Sobel D (1988) The Healing Brain: a Radical New Approach to Health Care. London: Macmillan.

Schor J (1991) The Overworked American: The Unexpected Decline of Leisure. New York: Basic Books.

Sigerist HE (1955) A History of Medicine. Vol. 1, Primitive and archaic medicine. New York: Oxford University Press.

Smith R (1987) Unemployment and Health: A Disaster and a Challenge. Oxford: Oxford University Press.

Stavrianos LS (1988) The World to 1500: A Global History. 4 edn. Englewood Cliffs NJ: Prentice-Hall.

Stevenson L (1987) Seven Theories of Human Nature. 2 edn. Oxford: Oxford University Press.

Virey JJ (1828) L'Hygiene Philosophique. Paris: Crochard.

Wharton WJL (ed.) (1893) Captain Cook's Journal during his First Voyage around the World made in HM Bark *Endeavour*. London: Eliot Stock, pp. 1768–71.

Wilcock AA (1993) A theory of the human need for occupation. Journal of Occupational Science: Australia 1(1): 17–24.

Wilcock AA (1998) An Occupational Perspective of Health. Thorofare, NJ: Slack Inc.

Wilcock AA, Dean P, Sturgul S (1993) Occupation and Health Survey. Unpublished data, School of Occupational Therapy, University of South Australia.

Wilcock AA, Darling K, Sholtz J, Siddall R, Snigg S, Stevens J, Van D'Arens (1991) An Exploratory Study of People's Perception and Experiences of Wellbeing. Unpublished data. School of Occupational Therapy, University of South Australia.

Wilcock AA, Van der Arend H, Darling K, Sholtz J, Siddall R, Snigg S, Stephens J (1998) An exploratory study of people's perceptions and experiences of well-being. British Journal of Occupational Therapy 61(2): 75–82.

Winefield A, Tiggerman M (1991) A longitudinal study of the psychological effects of unemployment and unsatisfactory employment on young adults. Journal of Applied Psychology 76(3): 424–31.

World Health Organisation (1946) Constitution of the World Health Organisation. New York: International Health Conference.

World Health Organisation (1978) Primary Health Care. Report of the International Conference on Primary Health Care, Alma-Ata, USSR.

World Health Organisation, Health and Welfare Canada, Canadian Public Health Association (1986) The Ottawa Charter for Health Promotion. Ottawa, Canada.

Yerxa EJ, Clark F, Frank G, Jackson J, Parham D, Pierce D, Stein C, Zemke R (1989) An introduction to occupational science: A foundation for occupational therapy in the 21st century. Occupational Therapy in Health Care, 6(4): 1–17.

Chapter 2
Purposeful activity

JENNIFER CREEK

Introduction

Occupational therapists claim that purposeful activity is both the goal of their interventions and one of the major tools they use. Christiansen (1991, p. 33) stated that 'The goal of occupational therapy is to prevent, remediate, or reduce dysfunction relating to occupational performance' and Ayres (1979, p. 183) described occupational therapy as 'a profession that employs a purposeful activity to help the client form adaptive responses'. It would, therefore, seem important that occupational therapists understand the nature of purposeful activity and its potential therapeutic effects.

Activity has been defined, for occupational therapists, as 'an integrated sequence of tasks which takes place on a specific occasion, during a finite period, for a particular purpose' (Hagedorn 1997, p. 143). This definition includes the idea of purposefulness as an integral part of activity.

The *Shorter Oxford English Dictionary* (Brown 1993) defined purposeful as: 'Having a purpose or meaning; indicating purpose; designed, intentional.' The word 'purpose' is given several definitions but the ones that are relevant in this context are: 'a thing to be done an object to be attained, an intention, an aim. The action or fact of intending to do something . . . the reason for which something is done or made, or for which it exists; the result or effect intended.'

According to these definitions, there are two aspects to purpose. First, purpose may reside in the intentions of the person carrying out the activity, or in the meaning he or she gives to it. Intention has been defined as 'the action or fact of intending to do a thing; what one intends to do, one's aim or design' (Brown 1993). For example, a young woman may do weight training in order to keep fit and because she enjoys the activity. She has two main purposes in carrying out the activity: fitness

16

and pleasure. Someone who leads an active life and neither feels the need to take more exercise nor finds pleasure in weight training would not find the activity purposeful. Second, purpose may exist in objects or activities irrespective of the person engaging with them. For example, washing up is for the purpose of cleanliness and hygiene, irrespective of who is carrying out the activity. Purpose may, of course, be found in both the person and the activity. For example, a woman doing the washing up may enjoy it, or may perceive washing up as part of her role as housewife. The purpose of the activity is still to produce clean dishes, but the woman's intention is to be a good housewife.

Occupational therapists and others have written much about purposeful activity and this chapter will begin by reviewing some of these writings in order to clarify what the term means. This will involve examining related concepts, including: volition, motivation, choice, autonomy, meaning and identity. From these concepts, a model or way of understanding purposeful activity will be constructed. This can be used to enhance our understanding of why the use of purposeful activities as treatment tools remains a vital part of occupational therapy intervention.

What is purposeful activity?

Most occupational therapy writers agree that the term purposeful activity refers to actions that are directed towards a goal or end result. For example, Kircher (1984, p. 165) offered this definition: 'Purposeful activity refers to tasks that are goal directed, focussing attention to an object or outcome.' Trombly (1995) spoke of the purpose of an activity being the goal. The goal of an activity influences the way that movements are organised and carried out, therefore it can be said that purpose organises behaviour towards a particular goal. Katz, Marcus, Weiss (1994, p. 200) pointed out that 'Purpose is not determined only by a finished product but by the process of doing.' So, the goal of a purposeful activity may be simply to do the activity, or may be to find a purpose. For example, I may feel bored and start a piece of embroidery in order to create a sense of purpose, a kind of 'purpose in progress'.

Some occupational therapy theorists have identified the location of purpose in the person carrying out the action, not in the activity itself. Breines (1984, p. 543) suggested that purposeful activities are 'unique constructions for individuals' and can only be defined in terms of the individual. Nelson (1988, p. 636) also suggested that 'the purpose of an occupational performance is always from the point of view of the actor. In other words, the term purpose is restricted to the goal orientation of the individual and does not refer to the goals of others'. This interpretation of purpose means that occupational therapists cannot give their patients purposeful activities but can only offer choices that allow people to follow their own directions. However, there may be confusion between purpose and meaning. Trombly (1995) separated the two concepts, locating purpose, or goal, in the activity and meaning in the person carrying out the activity. This conceptualisation means that occupational therapists can justly claim to provide their patients with purposeful activity, although the meaning that each person gives to the activity will be individual.

In order to understand activity, it is helpful to be clear about what is non-activity. The philosopher, Ginet (1990), divided activity into three types of actions:

• actions, or doing, which are voluntary exertions;
• non-actions, or not doing, which are voluntary inactivity;
• not actions, which are feelings, sensations, perceptions and involuntary movements, such as sneezing.

We can conclude that activity is any mental or physical action that is performed voluntarily, while non-activity is either voluntary inaction or involuntary action.

If all activities are voluntary, are they also purposeful? In order to answer this question, we need to explore the relationship between volition and purpose.

Volition and purpose

The *Shorter Oxford English Dictionary* (Brown 1993) defined volition as 'The action of consciously willing or resolving something; the making of a definite choice or decision regarding a course of action; exercise of the will.'

This definition assumes that volition itself is a mental action. Ginet (1990, p. 15) defined volition as 'the mental action with which one begins voluntary exertion of the body.' He emphasised that volition is not a precursor or trigger to action, or a separate action, but is a necessary component of voluntary exertion. Volition is the awareness, during an activity, of its being performed voluntarily. Ginet's conceptualisation of volition is a useful one for occupational therapists because it allows volition to be treated as a skill that is necessary for the performance of voluntary activity and which can be learned or improved. Ginet (1990) argued that all actions are intentional, that is, they begin with a purpose, even if the purpose changes during the course of the activity.

The action of volition can be detected by positron emission tomography (PET), a method of scanning the brain to measure cerebral activity. In a normal subject, the left dorsolateral prefrontal cortex is activated during the performance of intentional actions. It has also been reported that people with damage in this region of the brain exhibit a range of volitional disturbances (Dolan et al. 1993). These studies support strongly the notion that volition is a mental action and, furthermore, that it is focused in a particular region, or regions, of the brain. Activity in the prefrontal cortex appears to indicate 'inner representations of events in the future', that is, the imagination of goals and future events that must initiate voluntary action (Ingvar 1994, p. 9). Alterations in level of consciousness affect an individual's volitional capacity because 'conscious awareness is considered a prerequisite for wilful acts' (Ingvar 1994, p. 8). Low levels of awareness, such as sleepiness or boredom, and high levels of awareness, such as anxiety or pain, reduce the capacity to plan and carry out purposeful activities.

The philosopher, Ryle (1949), asserted that there is no evidence for the existence of volition and that the concept is both unnecessary and outdated. It is enough to be able to judge whether an action is voluntary or involuntary. Ryle argued that we can say an action is voluntary when a person does something he or she could have chosen not to do, but it does not follow that the action was purposeful. For example, 'to say that a laugh was voluntary is to say that the agent could have helped doing it . . . (but) we do not laugh on purpose.' Voluntariness is to do with opportunities and capacities, both of which are within the domain of concern of the occupational therapist, rather than with acts of will.

It is clear that volition is not a precursor or trigger to action, therefore, we require a different concept to understand what initiates purposeful activity. This concept is motivation. Motivation is 'The (conscious or unconscious) stimulus, incentive, motives etc., for action towards a goal . . . the factors giving purpose or direction to behaviour' (Brown 1993). The stimulus to action is experienced by the individual as a need. It may be triggered by external circumstances, such as the rapid approach of a car, which generates the need to run out of its path. A need may also arise from an internal circumstance, such as the feeling of hunger that triggers a need to eat. A third source of motivation and, occupational therapists would argue, a more basic one, is the intrinsic motivation to be active which is a characteristic of human beings. Sartre (1943) wrote that '. . . human reality does not exist first in order to act later; but for human reality, to be is to act and to cease to act is to cease to be.' The drive to act is a basic human need that must be satisfied.

If action is initiated by the stimulus of need, if people have the capacity to engage in activities that have purpose and meaning for them, and if they have opportunities to act, what influences their choice of activities? The next section deals with the concept of choice.

Choice and autonomy

It is in the nature of human beings to be active and most of their activities are not biologically programmed but are the result of series of choices. Some of these choices are small ones that are made on a regular basis, such as, 'shall I do some weeding or go window shopping for a couple of hours?' Other choices lead to time being structured for longer periods and so limit further choices. For example, when individuals make an occupational choice, such as becoming a full-time student, they accept that some of their time will be organised by the demands of that occupation, thus limiting the number of choices they to make on a day-to-day basis. The student will have to attend lectures and seminars at certain times during the week, there may be travelling time to and from the educational institution and he or she will have to do a certain amount of studying. Whether the individual makes many small choices each day, or has large blocks of time structured by previous occupational choices, the same factors influence why people choose to do certain activities rather than others, but the process of choice may be different.

Ginsberg, Ginsberg, Axelrad and Herma (1951) studied how people choose their main work occupation, finding that such an important decision is not made in one step but is the culmination of many smaller decisions made over many years. These could include what subjects to study at school, what leisure interests to pursue, whether to go on to higher education and which course to take. This long process of decision making allows the individual to accumulate knowledge of 'what he likes and what he dislikes; of what he does well and what he does poorly; the values which are meaningful to him and considerations which are unimportant' (Ginsberg et al. 1951, p. 29). The study concluded that four aspects of the self influence how people make occupational choices. These are: the individual's awareness of his own capacities; his interests; his personal goals and values, and his awareness of the time perspective of occupations. In addition, the opportunity for making a particular choice must be present.

What people may choose to do in the short or long term is partly influenced by the nature of the choices available. The range of choices is determined by social factors, such as public disapproval, and by the physical environment, such as the location of sport and leisure facilities. In order to choose to do something, the individual also has to be aware of what his choices are. This awareness includes knowing what activities are available and knowing how to access them. It also implies having the capacity to see opportunities for action and having enough information on which to base choices.

Choice may be limited by lack of awareness of one's own interests, capacities, values or goals, or by poor temporal awareness, or by lack of information about activities, or because of physical or social barriers. The capacity to make choices, or to exercise freedom of the will, is called autonomy. Barnitt (1993, p. 209) described autonomy as 'The freedom to decide, to act, to receive respect and retain dignity . . . to exercise choice and to be able to use the facts given.'

Gillon (1985) suggested that the ability to make choices depends on three types of autonomy. These are autonomy of thought, of will and of action. Autonomy of thought means being able to think for oneself, to have preferences and to make decisions. Autonomy of will means having the freedom to decide to do something or not to do something on the basis of one's deliberations. Autonomy of action is the capacity to act on the basis of deliberation and decisions made.

Autonomy is not an all or nothing capacity. Different people may have different degrees of autonomy and an individual's capacity for autonomous action is more limited at certain times of life, such as during infancy and periods of illness (O'Neill 1984). This suggests that autonomy has to be developed or learned by the growing child, therefore it can be developed or relearned at any time of life.

Being able to make and enact choices gives the individual a sense of control in her or his life, and quality of life appears to be at least partly dependent on having that sense of control. It is possible for an individual to have well-developed autonomy of thought and will even if his or her capacity for autonomous action is curtailed by disability. In such cases, disabled people may exercise their autonomy through others and so retain a feeling that they are controlling their own lives, for example by directing a helper to take them to the concert they want to attend.

So far, we have considered the nature of purpose, volition, motivation, choice and autonomy in an attempt to understand what is meant by purposeful activity. Another concept that has been mentioned but not yet discussed is meaning. The next section explores how the meanings that people give to their activities create a sense of purpose and how, in turn, activity helps to create meaning.

Meaning and identity

Meaning has been defined as 'that which is or is intended to be expressed or indicated by a sentence, word, dream, symbol, action, etc.' (Brown 1993). The word also incorporates the sense of significance or importance. So, when we talk about an activity having meaning for someone, we are saying that it is intentional and that it has some significance for the person carrying out the activity.

The activities that people choose to engage in have meaning for them, although that meaning may change over time. Primeau (1996) studied running and concluded that, as an activity, it 'has a social meaning derived from a shared cultural knowledge base' (p. 282) but also that 'the meaning and purposes of running may vary within the individual and across individuals' (p. 276).

Activities are not only ascribed meaning but they are also used to construct meaning. The Russian psychologist Vigotsky (1956) claimed that meaning does not direct activity but is created by it. It is through activity that people develop the neurological structures that underpin their cognitive processes. Zemke (1996) described how certain synaptic connections in the brain are strengthened during critical periods of learning to form cortical maps. These systems of neural linkages are unique to each individual and 'can determine the relative importance of external events according to internal values and schemes . . . (thus affecting) the selection of goals and purposeful action' (p. 167).

The meanings that people give to what they do come from two sources. They develop, in part, from the experiences of activity that the individual has had, and the associations and neural linkages that have been formed by those experiences. They also develop through interaction with other people, since all human activity takes place within the context of social relationships: 'Outside these relationships human activity simply does not exist' (Leont'ev 1978, p. 51). The social meaning of an activity is developed in the individual through learning the shared cultural knowledge base of the activity, that is, the acceptable techniques, context, materials, rules, sanctions and norms associated with the activity. This knowledge is shaped by feedback or reinforcement from others which gives a sense of the meaning and value of the activity as well as its structure or form. Each of us ascribes a meaning to the activities we engage in and those that we see others performing, and each of us is aware of at least some of the meanings that others give to those activities. The meaning of an activity is culturally specific in that the same activity will be given a different meaning and value in different cultures.

Breines (1995) developed a theory of occupational genesis that describes the nature of human activity in different ages and shows how activities develop to meet the needs of each culture. She demonstrated that the main activities of each age had meaning for people in terms of evolution, health and survival. The same activities may survive into later ages but their relevance will change.

People begin to make sense of the world, and to ascribe meanings to it, before they develop language. Simple or concrete concepts can be stored in non-linguistic cognitive schemas and communicated non-verbally (Bloom 1981). However, in order to understand and communicate more complex or abstract ideas, it is necessary to use language. The social meanings of activities are partly constructed and communicated through what is said and written about them. Bruner (1990), a psychologist, argued that the meanings placed on most actions in a social context are constructed by what the participants say about them before, during and after the action. For example, in the UK, smoking is widely reported to be damaging to the health of the smoker and those around him or her. The common social meaning of smoking in a public place is, therefore, a negative one.

In order for language to be used for communication, there has to be agreement between the speaker and listener on the meaning of the words used. This meaning comes from the intentions of the speaker, the socially agreed meaning of the words (how they are defined), the context of the communication and the understanding of the listener. Polatajko (1992) called the sharing of understanding and meaning within a culture 'framing' and said that 'Communication is based on the clear, precise sharing of meaning with another' (p. 191).

Shared meanings become internalised and help to create a sense of social and individual identity. If a person engages in an activity that is socially valued, such as driving a fast car, he will feel valued himself. If, on the other hand, an individual acts in a way that is given a low social value, such as begging for money in the street, he will internalise some of the meaning ascribed to that activity and feel worse about himself. This is a two-way process. When a person feels good about himself he is more likely to be active and to be successful in his activities. When someone has a low self-concept he is less likely to engage in activities and more likely to perform them badly.

Dennett (1991, p. 301) emphasised the importance of the language we use about ourselves in shaping identity: 'When you talk to yourself, you don't have to believe yourself in order for reactions to set in . . . so be careful what you say to yourself.' It is well known to cognitive psychologists that the self-talk people use when they are doing something affects the performance of the activity. The individual who is confident that he can perform competently, and who thinks that what he or she is doing is worthwhile, will perform better than the individual who doubts his or her capabilities or the value of the activity. People are more likely to choose to engage in activities that they can visualise themselves doing – activities that fit their self-image. In turn, the activities performed shape how people feel about themselves. Primeau (1996, pp. 283–4) described this process as 'an integration of self into a fuller sense of self'. Language acts as a mediator between self-image and activity in the construction of meaning.

Helfrich, Kielhofner and Mattingly (1994) studied the meanings that two people with severe mood disorders gave to their illness. The researchers looked at the relationship between what each person said about his or her illness and the individual's activities. They found that one person spoke of his disorder as a huge barrier to doing what he wants and described the tactics he uses to overcome it. He is not able to do all the activities he would do if he was not ill but he continues to work towards his personal goals. The other person described her illness as the end of all her hopes and opportunities. She has given up most of her previous activities and has become very inactive. In each case, the meaning that the individual gives to his or her illness, and the words used to describe it, shape what actions he or she takes to cope with it.

The first part of this chapter has attempted to clarify what is meant by purposeful activity and has discussed some of the concepts that are associated with it. From this discussion we can construct a model of purposeful activity that identifies the skills required for its performance and can act as a basis for occupational therapy intervention (Table 2.1).

Facilitating purposeful activity

The precursors of purposeful activity are consciousness, motivation and opportunity and these three factors remain present throughout the performance of the activity. They can also be enhanced by the activity, so they may become outcomes. The individual's level of consciousness will affect the extent to which the activity can be said to be purposeful. Motivation suggests need, or a drive to act, and may be intrinsic or extrinsic. Opportunities are features of the environment but it is necessary for the individual to be aware of them in order to act (Table 2.2).

In addition to these three precursors, the components of purposeful activity are capacities, volition, purpose, meaning and identity. Capacities include performance skills, autonomy of will and action, awareness of own capacities, temporal awareness and images of future events. Volition includes intentions, voluntary exertion and awareness of performing voluntarily. Purpose includes the object or goal of the activity and the purpose that is created by the activity, or purpose-in-progress. The meaning of an activity comes from its social context, from the past experiences of the individual and from the performance of the activity. The sense of identity created by the performance of an activity includes both social and individual identity. These five components

Table 2.1: Purposeful activity

Precursors	Components	Outcomes
Consciousness		
Motivation		
Opportunities		
	Capacities	
	Volition	
	Purpose	
	Meaning	
	Identity	
		Goals

Table 2.2: Precursors of purposeful activity

Consciousness	– level of awareness
Motivation	– intrinsic
	– extrinsic
Opportunities	– availability
	– awareness

Table 2.3: Components of purposeful activity

Capacities	– performance skills
	– autonomy of will and action
	– awareness of own capacities
	– temporal awareness
	– images of future events
Volition	– intentions
	– voluntary exertion
	– awareness of performing voluntarily
Purpose	– object or goal
	– purpose-in-progress
Meaning	– derives from social context
	– derives from past experience
	– created through performance
Identity	– social
	– individual

Table 2.4: The goals of occupational therapy intervention

Precursors to purposeful activity	• Enhancing consciousness
	• Providing opportunities
	• Providing extrinsic motivation
	• Accessing intrinsic motivation
Components of purposeful activity	• Teaching skills
	• Increasing competence
	• Rehearsing future events
	• Improving self-awareness
	• Enhancing the development of autonomy
	• Assisting in the construction of meaning
	• Helping to clarify values and intentions
	• Helping to identify personal goals
	• Offering purpose
	• Assisting with the development of volition
	• Helping to create identity
	• Respecting choices
	• Improving temporal orientation
Outcomes of purposeful activity	• Enabling achievement
	• Assisting towards the attainment of personal goals
	• Enhancing self image

remain present throughout the performance of the activity and may be enhanced by it, thus becoming outcomes as well as elements of purposeful activity (Table 2.3).

The main outcome of purposeful activity is the attainment of a goal or objective that can lead to a sense of achievement and an improved self-image.

Occupational therapy intervention

An individual's capacity for the performance of purposeful activity may be impaired if any of the necessary precursors is missing or if one or more of the additional components is lacking. Occupational therapy intervention may be targeted at any of the elements identified; for example, the therapist may wish to teach new skills or assist the client to identify personal goals. Taking each of the elements of purposeful activity identified in Tables 2.1, 2.2 and 2.3, we can see how the concept of purposeful activity informs the goals of occupational therapy intervention. These goals can be summarised as shown in Table 2.4.

In order to work towards the attainment of these goals, the occupational therapist provides activities that the patient finds interesting and worthwhile because they are purposeful and have meaning for her or him. The activities used as treatment media have a primary therapeutic purpose, but part of their potency is the multiple meanings they may hold for the patient. For example, a young woman with a learning disability made herself a cup of tea during therapy. 'For this client, making a cup of tea meant being able to do something for herself, to satisfy some of her own needs; it meant having success and a concrete end product that others would appreciate; it meant doing something that other young women in her culture took for granted; and it symbolised growing up and reducing her dependence on her parents' (Creek 1996, p. 129).

The occupational therapist should not assume that she understands the meanings that a particular activity has for a patient. Occupational therapists ascribe their own meanings to what the patient is doing and may give a high value to an activity, such as dressing independently, which is an important part of our professional role but is less important to the patient. It is necessary to ask people what an activity means to them and to listen to their stories without making judgements. However, the meaning of a therapeutic activity is not necessarily fully developed from the beginning of the intervention. Meaningfulness may be constructed through the performance of the activity and the ongoing discussion between the therapist and patient during the course of treatment (Trombly 1995).

Conclusion

This chapter has explored what is meant by purposeful activity and has identified the elements that make an activity purposeful. By identifying the components of purposeful activity, it has been possible to see what are the necessary conditions for its performance and what skills are required.

Purposeful activity is the goal of occupational therapy intervention. Most people take for granted their ability to engage in activities that have purpose and meaning for them. If the conditions are not right, they try to adapt the environment to provide the right conditions. If they lack skills, they try to acquire them or find a way of managing without them. People accept without question their right to act in ways that have purpose and meaning for them, therefore the goal of occupational therapy is readily comprehensible and acceptable.

Purposeful activity is also a major tool of intervention for occupational therapists but this can be more problematic. It is easy to forget that the activities in which most people engage without thought are not simple but require a complex range of conditions and skills. To provide an activity to pass time or to exercise a limb is not very difficult, but to enable an individual to engage in an activity that has purpose and meaning for her or him, and which will assist in the development of performance skills, is the highest art of the occupational therapist.

References

Ayres AJ (1979) Sensory Integration and the Child. Los Angeles: Western Psychological Services.

Barnitt R (1993) What gives you sleepless nights? Ethical practice in occupational therapy. British Journal of Occupational Therapy 56(6): 207–12.

Bloom AH (1981) The Linguistic Shaping of Thought: a Study in the Impact of Language in Thinking in China and the West. Hillsdale NJ: Lawrence Erlbaum.

Bruner J (1990) Acts of Meaning. Cambridge MA: Harvard University Press.

Breines EB (1984) The issue is an attempt to define purposeful activity. American Journal of Occupational Therapy 38(8): 543–4.

Breines EB (1995) Occupational therapy activities from clay to computers: theory and practice. Philadelphia PA: FA Davis.

Brown L (ed.) (1993) The New Shorter Oxford English Dictionary. Oxford: Clarendon Press.

Christiansen C (1991) Occupational therapy intervention for life performance. In Christiansen C, Baum C (eds) Occupational Therapy: Overcoming Human Performance Deficits. Thorofare NJ: Slack.

Creek J (1996) Making a cup of tea as an honours degree subject. British Journal of Occupational Therapy 59(3): 128–30.

Dennett DC (1991) Consciousness Explained. London: Penguin.

Dolan RJ, Bench CJ, Liddle PF, Friston KJ, Frith CD, Grasby PM, Frackowiak RSJ (1993) Dorsolateral prefrontal cortex dysfunction in the major psychoses; symptom or disease specificity? Journal of Neurosurgery and Psychiatry 56: 1290–4.

Gillon R (1985) Autonomy and the principle of respect for autonomy. British Medical Journal 290: 1806–8.

Ginet C (1990) On Action. Cambridge: Cambridge University Press.

Ginsberg E, Ginsberg SW, Axelrad S, Herma JL (1951) Occupational choice: an approach to a general theory. New York: Columbia University Press.

Hagedorn R (1997) Foundations for Practice in Occupational Therapy, 2 edn. Edinburgh: Churchill Livingstone.

Helfrich C, Kielhofner G, Mattingly C (1994) Volition as narrative: understanding motivation in chronic illness. American Journal of Occupational Therapy 48(4): 311–17.

Ingvar DA (1994) The will of the brain: cerebral correlates of willful acts. Journal of Theoretical Biology 171(1): 7–12.

Katz N, Marcus S, Weiss P (1994) Purposeful activity in physical rehabilitation. Critical Reviews in Physical and Rehabilitation Medicine 6(2): 199–218.

Kircher MA (1984) Motivation as a factor of perceived exertion in purposeful versus nonpurposeful activity. American Journal of Occupational Therapy 38(3): 165–70.

Leont'ev AN (1978) Activity, Consciousness and Personality. New York: Prentice-Hall.

Nelson DL (1988) Occupation: form and performance. American Journal of Occupational Therapy 42(10): 633–41.

O'Neill O (1984) Paternalism and partial autonomy. Journal of Medical Ethics 10: 173–8.

Primeau LA (1996) Running as an occupation: multiple meanings and purposes. In Zemke R, Clark F (eds) Occupational Science: the Evolving Discipline. Philadelphia: FA Davis.

Polatajko HJ (1992) Naming and framing occupational therapy: a lecture dedicated to the life of Nancy B. Canadian Journal of Occupational Therapy 59(4):189–99.

Ryle G (1949/1990) The concept of mind. Harmondsworth: Penguin.

Sartre JP (1943) (trans. Barnes HE 1966) Being and Nothingness. London: Methuen.

Trombly CA (1995) Occupation: purposefulness and meaningfulness as therapeutic mechanisms. American Journal of Occupational Therapy 49(10): 960–72.

Vigotsky LS (1956) Collected Psychological Works. Moscow.

Zemke R (1996) Brain, Mind and Meaning. In Zemke R, Clark F (eds) Occupational Science: The Evolving Discipline. Philadelphia: FA Davis.

Chapter 3
Shifting ground or sifting sand?

MARY JENKINS

'Criticism and critical discussion are our only means of getting nearer to the truth.' (Popper 1965, p. 151)

Introduction

This chapter is based on my own work into practice effectiveness in occupational therapy. It is intended to provide a critical review of my work and that of other writers in the field. This issue of criticism is a key one. According to the *Concise Oxford Dictionary* it can mean 'finding fault, censure' but it can also mean 'an article, essay, etc., expressing or containing an analytical evaluation of something.' The latter meaning would seem to incorporate the notion of critical thinking for the purpose of informing or educating. This is appealing; the intention is to open up the subject matter for discussion, for exploration, for perusal and even for truth, as Popper (1965) implied. The outcome of this process should be a move towards a synopsis of my own concept of practice effectiveness and the ramifications that presents.

Jenkins' concept of practice effectiveness

This concept was derived from research findings that suggested that occupational therapy is a personal service where practice is concerned with situational problems and with the need for interactants – that is, clients and practitioners – to generate personally relevant theory to understand these problems (Jenkins 1994a). The profession of occupational therapy is a personalised service contiguous with clients' lifeworld contexts.

Before continuing, it is important that the concept of 'lifeworld contexts' is explained. This does not denote a physical environment, as some readers have understood it, but rather clients' lifeworld contexts describe where they are at that point in time, in being not in place. Crucially, occupational therapy has a pragmatic orientation and rests on contact and first-hand experiences with clients and their worlds. It is indisputably person focused. Practice does not revolve around abstract principles, or abstractions, as Whitehead referred to them when he said 'Professional education produces minds in a groove. Now to be mentally in a groove is to live contemplating a given set of abstractions . . . but there is no groove of abstraction which is adequate for the comprehension of human life' (Whitehead 1926, p. 282–3). Rather, practice revolves around real-life situations. As one speech and language therapist described it: 'They [occupational therapists] do not simply look at the stroke patient, the actual presenting symptoms, they actually look at the patient, where they're coming from and where they're going to' (Jenkins and Brotherton 1995b, p. 332).

This dimension of wholeness, of total being, has the immediate effect of contextualising the client in his or her own lived-in reality which, in essence, becomes the actual situation of practice, the site according to Lave 'of the most powerful knowledgeability of people' (1988, p. 14). This situatedness, its potency and some notion of lifeworld context, is further explained by reporting the critical incident that the above-mentioned therapist went on to relate:

> My mum has a severe stroke. At the beginning they [occupational therapists] got her the most independent that she could be in that they found what she really wanted, she needed. She always enjoyed it and the occupational therapist, especially in the early stages, had really good fun with her. As well she explained to her and gave reasons why she couldn't do the things that she thought she would be able to do and why she'd come so far and also gave what she would possibly expect in the future and where she would like to see her going and that kind of thing. At this stage it's good in that they've been working with other agencies and with my father who found it quite difficult to accept so they involved him in the therapy, working out the best regarding the house, adaptations, etc.' (Jenkins and Brotherton 1995b, p. 333)

The consensus is that intervention is good when client and practitioner listen to each other. The above story demonstrates an interactive process that is not only explicit in the practitioner and client experience but is also evidenced in the way treatment is integrated into the situation of the individual, the family and their wider life context. It also presents a practice in which interactants share and develop knowledge through their mutual experience. There is a oneness about this similar to Fuller's idea of singleness that consists of 'two sides reciprocally entering into one another's lives' (1983, p. 384).

To establish further the propriety of the practice environment for learning, and to produce *in vivo* this process of inter-experience, I cite the following discourse between client and practitioner (P – practitioner, C – client):

P: It's sore?
C: It is.
P: Is it your knee that's sore?
C: It's there and just comes right round there.
P: Aye.
C: This knee, there's not a lot of muscle in this knee now since I've taken that: that's a year and a half, 2 years ago.
P: Aye
C: Not a lot of muscle, this knee's always sore.
P: You see what happens when you've got a painful hip, you're trying to save that leg and protect it and you don't use it as much and often all the muscles weaken and then when you had your hip replaced and a new one put in, you've to try and strengthen up that leg again but it's sore, it's painful . . .
C: Yeah.
P: And it takes maybe six months or longer to get that knee fully strengthened again.
C: Yes, I agree with you. (Jenkins et al. 1994, p. 301)

The intercourse that exists here, when practitioner and client show this degree of reciprocity and understanding, is the kernel of practice effectiveness as it is described in this chapter. This level of intimacy in communication predisposes learning and is particularly relevant to occupational therapists given their involvement in the everyday events of clients' lives and the events that matter to them. As Bockoven remarked: 'The occupational therapist's inborn respect for the realities of life, for the real tasks of living and for the time it takes the individual to do the tasks' (1971, p. 225). The person–environment relationship becomes a fitting breeding ground for the generation of knowledge and ultimately practice effectiveness.

Legitimate peripheral participation perspective

The findings concur with Lave and Wenger's legitimate peripheral participation perspective (1989) and constitute a theoretical framework for occupational therapy practice (Jenkins and Brotherton 1995c). The picture is one of a practice where interrelationships between practitioner and client, between client and his or her lifeworld context, between practitioner and his or her professional world context are pivotal.

The three contexts interrelate and together constitute the practice world, urging mutual ownership of problems and resolution. The outcome of this dynamic situation is learning on the part of the client and on the part of the practitioner that is actualised in personal and professional growth. This does not happen when there are blockages in any of the three relationships, as shown in the following examples related by practising occupational therapists.

1. Between practitioner and client

I remember this lady who had a stroke, she was very young, would have been 34: she had a very dense stroke and the OT told her that her arm would never be any good to her. I know she had to face up to this but I don't think she should have been told that way. I think she should have been told 'It may take a long time'. For a while she didn't do anything – she refused to come to outpatient clinic . . . Eventually it ended up her husband left her and she had to cope with all the children – she had four – but I felt it could have been approached differently, it may have helped. But she was told straight out it's not getting any better. (Jenkins and Brotherton 1995b, p. 335)

2. Between client and his or her lifeworld context

You can be the perfect occupational therapist. You can do every-thing by the book, you can throw everything at them but to me if the patient isn't interested, has lost all will to live or thinks 'This is it for the rest of my life'. I've seen it happen. If the patient cannot grasp what you're about or what you want to do, there is no point in going on, is there? (Jenkins and Brotherton 1995b, p. 334)

3. Between practitioner and professional world context

I was doing a placement in a day hospital where there were several pieces of equipment; an OB arm, a bicycle, a treadle sewing machine. I'm sure there were one or two other things: everyone who came in, regardless of disease, age, sex, went from one to the other. None of them were used as purposeful activity, so people just went from one to the other. It included the men, big farmers coming in and operating the treadle sewing machine, but it also included the young MS patients coming in doing the same as everyone else. It was neither disease oriented nor patient oriented: it must have been equipment oriented. (Jenkins 1995b, p. 334)

The potency of all these practice situations is transparent. They do happen but they do not have to, given the propriety of the situation for progress and given that each interactant accepts and owns their responsibility for moving forward. Inclusivity is vital and it is this factor that, in my view, makes the findings regarding practice effectiveness so relevant in this present day of change in health care.

Practice in transition

There are a number of variables that have influenced a worldwide restructuring of health services and a redesigning of care and delivery. The move is driven by financial considerations and a consumerist philosophy that seeks to redefine the roles of protagonists in healthcare – the patient and the professional.

In the UK, the change has been assisted by Government in reforming the National Health Service (NHS) as a business organisation. The shift from a baseline of socialised health care towards a market economy was begun with the implementation of Griffiths' recommendations in 1984 and was fully realised in the NHS reforms instigated by the then Prime Minister, Margaret Thatcher, and sanctioned via the NHS and Community Care Act 1990.

The reason for the transformation is clearly stated in 'Working for Patients' (DOH 1989, paragraphs 1:15 and 1:16):

> If the NHS is to provide the best service it can for its patients it must make the best use of resources available to it. The quest for value for money must be an essential element in its work. Those who take decisions that involve spending money must be accountable for that spending. Equally, those who are responsible for managing the service must be able to influence the way in which its resources are used.

A definitive feature of the reforms is the development of health authorities and, in Northern Ireland, health and social services boards, as purchasers and organisers of care, and professionals as providers of that care. The step is towards 'a partnership – between central and local government, between health and social services, between government and the private and voluntary sectors, between professionals and individuals – to the benefit of those in need' (Griffiths 1988, p. 25) and away from a hierarchical system controlled by doctors and medical professionals where finance was not a factor (Ham 1981; Hunter 1991) The decentralisation of power is ongoing and is bringing with it a re-ordering of roles – a timely event, some have remarked, given that the transition is stimulated not only by Government thinking, but by public and professional challenges.

The traditional role of medicine

The legitimacy of medical autocracy derives from the discovery and acceptance of germ theory, which marked the beginning of modern biomedicine (Allan and Hall 1988). It revolutionised the age-old profession by providing a scientific rationale for the continued commitment to the Cartesian belief in the separateness of mind and body, and ensured its status over patients and other health care occupations. A facilitating factor is that medical authority has been State sustained and circumscribed both in Britain (Larkin 1988) and in America (Preston 1982).

In the UK, initially, medical dominance was assured by State registration through the 1858 Medical Act and then the founding of the Ministry of Health in 1918, which intensified an alliance that culminated in doctors' ascendancy as principal players in the NHS from its inception in 1948. Elston summed up their position: 'Far from being proletarianised by accepting salaried status, consultants have enjoyed great power and authority under this system. NHS hospitals have been ruled, not by a single manager, but by the collective power of individual medical preference' (1993, p. 47). The scenario was repeated worldwide. The medical world had a monopoly on explaining sickness in terms of disease, the focus was the body whereas the personal, social and cultural contexts became irrelevant. The sick person became objectified and subordinate, as described by Friedson (1970):

> On entering the professional domain, however, due process is lost. The citizen is expected to give up all but the most humble rights, to put himself into the hands of the expert and trust his judgement and good intentions. He is expected to take a role that is akin to that of a house pet, or a child, dependent on the benevolence and knowledgeability of the adult caretaker. (p. 355)

This view of the power of the medical profession was shared by Parsons (1951) who extends it to all the professions. It is important to note the two assumptions on which Parsons' notion of professional behaviour is founded. First, the patient has a need for technical services because he does not know what is the matter or what to do about it, nor does he control the necessary facilities; second, the doctor is a technical expert who by special training and experience is qualified to help the patient (1951). Acceptance of this asymmetric relationship confers professional authority and legitimises the existence of the knowledge gap, in addition to justifying the patient's trust and obedience. Interestingly, this was not always the case. During the time of Hippocrates, in the fourth century BC, medicine was holistic, having what Cassel (1964) called a panenvironmental focus, more akin to the ecological view of today, which stresses wholeness, quality of life, the environment and the interactions among these factors.

Although Hippocrates laid down his principles of medical law/medicine 400 years before the birth of Christ, they are still relevant today in that they were assumed into the Hippocratic oath which graduating medical students have taken since the nineteenth century. The oath describes medicine as an art first and foremost: 'To reckon him who taught me this art equally dear to me as my parents . . .With purity, and with holiness I will pass my life and practise my art' (World Books 1977, p. 227)

In Hippocrates' view the goal of the physician was the care of the patient, 'For where there is the love of man, there is also love of the Art' (p. 227). His practice was basically situational, treating his patients with proper diet, fresh air, change in climate and attention to habits and living conditions. Medicine as an art viewed man as an individual and worked with him in context to better his situation. Medicine as a science seems to have swept away humaneness, or has had it swept away by the persuasiveness of technocratic logic that separates out the disease from the person, treating it as a self-contained entity. Cassell noted the process:

> The story of an illness – the patient's history – has two protagonists, the body and the person. By careful questioning it is possible to separate out the facts that speak of disturbed bodily functioning, the patho-physiology that gives you the diagnosis. To do this, the facts about the body's dysfunction must be separated from the meanings that the patient has attached to them. Skilful physicians have been doing this for ages. All too often, however, the personal meanings are then discarded. With them go the doctor's opportunity to know who the patient is. (1985, p. 108)

Adherence to the biomedical model of care brings with it a mindset that holds the dependency of the patient and the superordinancy of the professional as supreme. This fact was acknowledged by Brown (1979) when he confirmed that medicine's power in the USA had become so politicised that it had ensured the elimination of other, less disease-oriented, professions. Allan and Hall (1988) pinpointed its effect there on the nursing profession, seeing dehumanisation as the greatest problem and noting that medicine kills the disease while ignoring the cost to the person. Similar concerns were reiterated by Canadian writers Hewa and Hetherington in their pointedly named article 'Specialists without spirit: crisis in the nursing profession'. They concluded that healthcare services are increasingly devoid of human relations, and 'individual patients are treated without regard for psychological, social and cultural differences . . . Psychology, spirituality and emotions are not regarded as important aspects of medicine, nor are they part of medical jargon' (1990, p. 181). Yet these very same sentiments were being voiced within the medical profession as long ago as 1926, when Crookshank referred in the *Lancet* to the clinical method 'that gives excellent schemes for the physical examination of the patient whilst strangely ignoring, almost completely, the psychical' (p. 941). Similar observations were made a year later by Harvard Physician FW Peabody, in the *Journal of the American Medical Association* (1922):

> The most common criticism made at present by older practitioners is that younger graduates have been taught a great deal about the mechanisms of disease but very little about the practice of medicine – or to put it more bluntly, they are too scientific and do not know how to take care of patients (cited by Culliton 1984, p. 420).

The propensity of the scientific approach to concentrate on the symptoms of disease rather than the person was realised quickly but its invasiveness has continued to grow. Yerxa (1980) fittingly described the journey from humanism to scientism in a society dominated by technique when she said, 'The end product of the marriage between modern science and technology that attempts to control nature, seemingly as an expression of man's will to power but that itself appears to be increasingly in control of humanity' (p. 530). There is no doubt that this has happened in the process of scientific rationalisation of health care and it was a natural consequence, as Weber advised (1958). There is a danger that those who use the scientific rationale are unaware of its dehumanising nature and have not, even in the face of sharp criticism and convincing arguments, succeeded in applying it in a way that overcomes this deficiency. We have allowed technological development to supersede the metaphysical aspects of human existence yet, in doing so, have still not achieved true rationalisation, that is, the eradication of the consequences of our own irrational behaviour, either by complementary corrective strategies or by choosing alternative courses of action (Weber 1964 in Lasserman and Velody 1989). Weber, in his lecture 'Science as a Vocation' to students of Munich University in 1917, forecast the present position:

> The fate of our age, with its characteristic rationalisation and intellectualisation and above all the disenchantment of the world, is that the ultimate most sublime values have withdrawn from public life, either into the transcendental realm of mystical life or into the brotherhood of immediate personal human relations (in Lasserman and Velody 1989, p. 175).

It seems that the dehumanisation of health services is widespread, and yet it is the acknowledgement of direct human experience which lifts professional practice from the mundane to the vital. The next section describes some alternative approaches to the professional – patient relationship.

The art of caring

Given the insight of science itself into its practice, it would be expected that rational thought would have urged a move towards ensuring an appreciation of the patient as a whole. Engel and Balint are medical personnel who have attempted to do this, Engel by submitting an alternative approach, the biopsychosocial model, and Balint by complementing the traditional medical approach with clinical group discussions. Engel (1977) introduced systems theory – an approach that integrates biological, psychological and social information of the patient into the picture of sickness – so involving the organic, personal and interpersonal milieux. Rather than reducing the story, systems theory enlarges it until all significant relationships are included. It is not prescriptive and is conceived by traditionalists to lack credibility because of its dependence on person input from both the practitioner and the client.

Balint, a psychoanalyst whose father was a general practitioner in Hungary, realised the inadequacies of the traditional method for reaching any deep understanding of the patient's illness. He believed the need was to listen, not to ask questions (the technique of the clinical method). He developed the concepts of attentive listening and responding to a patient's 'offers' as ways of understanding his illness. Additionally, such discussions allow doctors to look at their own practice relationships, consider their own roles in these and, through time, increase their own self-awareness. As Balint put it, 'it invariably also entails a limited, though considerable, change in the doctor's personality' (Balint 1957, p. 59).

The overall aim of both approaches is to assist practitioners to listen to their patients, to perceive their needs and understand their sufferings, because the conventional biomedical model, though having a monopoly on explaining illness, does not do so. It is too doctor-centred. Mishler (1984) insisted that medical practice should be patient-centred, as only patients' lifeworld contexts of meaning can form the basis for understanding, diagnosing and treating their problems. In this model, communication rather than inquisition becomes the central activity of the encounter and, although the biopsychosocial model, as described by Engel, has been slow to gain acceptance, the techniques used in the model have been shown to be effective in gaining the patient's co-operation and participation in treatment regimes and therapy programmes.

Kleinman, Eisenberg and Good (1978) argued for the establishment of a therapeutic alliance. Their work subscribes to a negotiation model in which empathy is critical. 'Indeed we regard empathy as so crucial to the negotiation model that it is unlikely that the elicitation of the patient's model and subsequent negotiation is possible without an affective bond between doctor and patient' (Katon and Kleinman 1981, p. 266). By evoking a patient's attitudes and beliefs about disease and treatment there is more likely to be a successful outcome and by neglecting these there is more likelihood of non-compliance, dissatisfaction, litigation and distrust. The development of mutual trust and clinical negotiation seems central (Bernarde and Mayerson 1978; Brody 1980; Lazare, Eissenthal and Wasserman 1975; Stewart 1984). Stewart's work, in particular, found an association between patient satisfaction and the opportunity to share opinions during the interview, while Bernarde and Mayerson (1978) found an association between patient/practitioner respect, eye contact, question answering and, importantly, the physician's emotional sensitivity, a potent ingredient as displayed in Kleinman's work. This factor is one that throws open to question the formal professional stance as advanced by the Parsonian concept of professionalism and perpetuated by the biomedical approach. The legitimacy of this institutionalised model of professional behaviour has to be queried and thought should be given to equalising the experience. Mutuality, evidently, is no longer only something voiced by occupational therapists alone (Bockoven 1971; Englehardt 1977; Mocellin 1988; Peloquin 1991; Yerxa 1967). It is acknowledged as part of a caring relationship 'which makes the patient feel valued as an individual, offers him understanding and empathy and serves to increase his sense of identity and integrity' (Williams 1993, p. 13).

Barbara Korsh has been researching the doctor–patient relationship since the 1960s, using an adapted version of Bale's interaction process analysis (Bale 1980 in Stewart and Roter 1989), originally developed for assessing counselling interactions. She said clearly that:

> Our patients have shown us that they want more knowledge about health and a more active part in doctor–patient communication. Thus the doctor–patient relationship is shifting more and more in the direction of interactions and egalitarian participation, centring on the patient as a person, taking into account his individuality and cultural strengths and weaknesses' (in Stewart and Roter 1989, p. 250)

Occupational therapy in transition

These values have been held by occupational therapists since the beginning of the profession, as verified by Meyer, a psychiatrist, who was a prominent pioneer of occupational therapy and who articulated this philosophy as early as 1922:

The evolution of occupational therapy represents to me a very important manifestation of a very general gain in human philosophy. The most important fact in the progress lay undoubtedly in the newer conceptions of mental problems of living, and not merely diseases of a structural and toxic nature on the one hand or of a final lasting constitutional disorder on the other. (Meyer 1922, p. 4)

Occupational therapy was born out of these convictions and won its place initially because some physicians saw the advantages of moral treatment – that through gainful occupations and human interplay persons could be assisted towards health. Around this same time Dewey, the educationalist, was also extolling the virtues of occupations. Apart from sense training and discipline in thought, he noted that they offered 'a spirit of free communication, of interchange of ideas, suggestions, results . . .' (Dewey 1900, pp. 15–16). For the purposes of credibility and employability, occupational therapy pioneers courted the medical profession. The prominence of its influence in the formative and developmental stage of occupational therapy is demonstrated in these words, voiced by Dr C Charles Burlingame and imparted by Slagle at a conference on occupational therapy held in London, July 11 1934:

What is an occupational therapist? She is that newer medical specialist who takes the joy out of invalidism . . . The duties of this new medical specialist begin at the earliest possible moment, before enforced idleness has started to do permanent damage to the mind and body of the ill person. It is to her that the doctor gives detailed instruction as to what use is to be made of the resources of the patient's mind and body which are still available.

Where is the occupational therapist? Wherever there are doctors there should be an occupational therapist. Who is the occupational therapist? – a highly trained medical assistant, possessed of imaginative ability and cultural background. (1934, p. 290–1)

The marriage seemed solid, yet the coupling of a discipline founded and developed on humanistic principles with one rooted in biomedicine and scientism must eventually lead to controversy. This has indeed happened, to the point that occupational therapy has had to re-establish itself as a discipline wherein client-centredness is fundamental to its practice. The demand has been evident for some time, not only among occupational therapists but also in the medical profession itself. Indeed, Bockoven wrote, in 1971: 'It is time for occupational therapists to listen to the idea that their profession has been the child of medicine long enough and to consider that it is ready to go off on its own as the next step toward full maturity and full social effectiveness' (p. 224). Like any divorce, it has not been easy and the profession has faced internal struggles. It would now, however, seem to be arriving at the point where it can back up its own theories of occupation with research.

The Canadian Association of Occupational Therapists was alone in taking the person-centred approach as its focus, even during those years of confusion caused by attempts to dance to the same tune as medicine, when it was clear that we could not. It may be that occupational therapists in other countries took for granted that client-centredness is integral to our practice and so failed to discuss or write about it. The person-centred approach is an essential ingredient of situated learning and thence effective practice. One client described it as: 'You are coming to talk to the soul of the person, whereas others have dealt with the leg, or whatever. You know you are getting to the inner person' (Jenkins 1994a, p. 240).

The importance of sensitivity is a factor, which Rogers recognised early on in his career in psychotherapy, and of which he said:

> It involves being sensitive, moment to moment, to the changing felt meanings which flow in this other person, to the fear or rage or tenderness or confusion or whatever that he/she is experiencing. It means temporarily living in his/her life, moving about it delicately without malign judgements, sensing meaning of which he/she is scarcely aware . . . (in Thorne 1992, p. 142)

The centrality of sensitivity in effective counselling is undisputed. The transaction is two way, even if sometimes only by accommodation. The statement by Watzlawick et al. (1967, p. 49) that 'one cannot not communicate' is true because we say so much through body language, as LaCrosse's (1975) work confirms. Behaviours, such as smiles, nods and leaning forward 20 degrees, increase the client's perception of the practitioner's warmth, interest, effectiveness and concern. It would appear that we, as a profession, have made a circular trip, a cycle of life, a life cycle even.

Democracy in practice

Occupational therapy has, in effect, come back to where we started from, as indeed has medicine, and the feeling is one of trustworthiness of fit because we are, after all, fiduciaries. As fiduciaries, we hold in trust those services the patient needs and the education and training the student must have. We do not own the services we provide, we simply serve and are as accountable to our clients as to our profession and peer professions. Zimmerman made the comment some years ago, 'If health care is to be humanised, we as providers must first be persons ourselves' (1974, p. 467). We must be open and inviting to clients, their concerns and feelings, as they must be open to us, to our ideas and our notions. The relationship centres on interpersonal dependencies within the practice environment that allow practitioner and client to enter into what Fuller (1983) terms 'a relationship of knowing.'

Practice that is co-determined by client and practitioner is more effective than professional-led practice. This contention is supported by my own research findings and those of others (for example, Inui and Carter 1985; Roter, Hall and Katz 1988; Wasserman and Inui 1983). The ramifications are a rethinking of the professional's input and impact that, until now, has been based on 'expert' knowledge. Yet, we have been arguing that the most important practitioner ingredient in effective practice is the 'self' of the professional – not his or her technical knowledge, which Parsons (1951) claimed for the professional, but a self which has been formed in the course of experiential relationships in practice. The most important client ingredient is his knowledge of self and, as if in direct opposition to Parsons, it has been demonstrated that clients do know that something is the matter, they do have an opinion as to how they can work to better the situation and, although they do not have control over 'the necessary facilities', their input is vital to any satisfactory resolution. It has been shown that only where professional and client act together in formulating the end and the means of service provision, when they have equal say and share in the practice event, is best practice actualised or realised.

One client expressed it in these words: 'For me it was finding the place that I could achieve in life. You kept moving onto the next until I moved onto university which is fairly challenging to me' (Jenkins 1994a, p. 368) and 'it's something that no-one else applies. It moves slightly outside the medical treatment, it moves you into society' (Jenkins and Brotherton 1995b, p. 332).

In democratising the intervention, are we dismissing the relevance of professionalism or can we address it in such a way that it retains its worth in the service of the individual?

There is need within professionalism to achieve a relationship that allows questioning, exchange of information, mutual understanding and agreement on the mode of treatment and shared plans for meeting long-term treatment goals. I cannot accept that we should conform to Illich's concept of 'disabling' professions (1972). The term 'disabling professions' is ironic and almost perverse and yet his perception of professionalism is justified or, at least, has some worth as the previous arguments show. However, professions are not types of occupations but historical forms of controlling occupations. They act to determine how work should be done and by whom, as well as claiming special, incommunicable authority to decide not just the way things are to be but also the reasons why their services are mandatory. They are almost union-like; the image of professionalism can be unsettling:

> professionals are the people who guide us through life's crises, make decisions about our bodies, our children, ourselves. They write letters to each other about us and wield power over us . . . I hate it [professionalism] because it is elitist and divisive. It simultaneously creates an illusion of superiority and coerces people into complying with unreasonable demands . . . It creates an atmosphere of paternalism, of bounty given with dignity and received with submissive gratitude. (Windsor 1991, p. 5)

Conclusion

It would seem that people have felt used and abused by professionals long enough – it is time for action. The caveat will no longer be, 'I act, you act, they act', as Spiegal (1973) said of professional groups. Rather, it will be 'we act'. The turn around is close to Holler's belief that 'what the future holds for us depends on what we hold for the future' (in Bruhn 1987, p. 116). The question, given this new situation, is 'are we ready for democratic professionalism, so removing the element of inequality that traditional professionalism seems to expound?' Jenkins' concept of practice effectiveness utilises the notion of partnership and participation without compromising either professional or client autonomy. It urges a change in the professional's role, a change in professionalism and, most specifically, says that the knowledge of the profession which best informs practice is indeed integral to that practice (Jenkins 1994b, 1995c). This is not a disavowal of professional knowledge but rather an acknowledgement that it can be enhanced in collaboration with clients when approaches to care and recovery are negotiated rather than imposed. The situation is one that Wilding was advancing in 1982: 'They [the professions] have to be persuaded of the advantages of a partnership relationship both for themselves and for their clientele' (p. 144). Democratic professionalism concentrates on the individuality of the person receiving the service. It rests on the dynamics of the interaction and pivots on the ability of the professional to use his or her knowledge with and for the client rather than over and against him or her. It rests on:

- collaboration with clients, significant others and carers in treatment;
- the essence of appreciating client input and his/her knowledge in the formulation of treatment programmes;
- the existence of a two-way communication process which acknowledges the client's viewpoint fully, rather than incidentally and indifferently. (Jenkins 1994b, p. 131).

The bonus of this 'person approach' is that it fosters the empowerment of clients to function better in their real-life situations and enables practitioners to build their professional practice knowledge through experiencing this lived-in world. The naming and framing of problems is a mutual act where knowledge growth and understanding evolve and where there is a democracy in play. Unlike Schön's (1987) notion of practice effectiveness, naming and framing is owned by both interactants. It is not solely a characteristic of the professional.

The situation presupposes the centrality of the service ethic, to which Hugman (1991) refers, and has regard for love that was, after all, a focus of the early Greek medical practitioners and the first occupational therapists: 'It is not enough to give a patient something to do with his hands. You must reach for the heart as well as the hands. It's the heart that really does the healing' (Carlova and Ruggles 1946, pp. 249–50). More recently, Vanier spoke of the significance of love for the client: 'He must discover he is loved and important to someone. Only then will he discover he is worthwhile and only then will his confusion turn to peace' (1992, p. 259–60).

In this new, ecologically oriented consumerist society, if it is reasonable to accept Allan and Hall's vision of the health practitioner as 'one who acts as a consultant to the client for goal-setting and advice on health practices to achieve self care' (1988, p. 32), then it is reasonable to accept democratic professionalism and the notion that practice effectiveness is a determinant of practice relationships.

References

Allan JD, Hall BA (1988) Challenging the focus on technology: a critique of the medical model in a changing health care system. Advances in Nursing Science 10(3): 22–34.

Bale RF (1950) Interaction Process Analysis. Cambridge: Addison Wesley.

Balint M (1961) The other part of medicine. Lancet 1: 40–2.

Bernarde MA, Mayerson EW (1978) Patient–physician negotiation. Journal of the American Medical Association 239: 1413–15.

Bockoven JS (1971) Legacy of moral treatment – 1800–1910. American Journal of Occupational Therapy 25(5): 223–35.

Brody DS (1980) The patient's role in clinical decision-making. Annals of Internal Medicine 93: 718–22.

Brown RGS (1979) Reorganizing the National Health Service: a case study in administrative change. Oxford: Blackwell.

Bruhn JG (1987) The changing limits of professionalism in allied health. Journal of Allied Health (May): 111–18.

Carlova J, Ruggles O (1946) The Healing Heart. New York: Messner.

Cassel J (1964) Social science theory as a source of hypotheses in epidemiological research. American Journal of Public Health 54: 1482–8.

Cassell EJ (1985) Talking with Patients. Volume 2: Clinical Technique. Cambridge MA: MIT Press.

Crookshank FG (1926) The theory of diagnosis. Lancet 2: 939–42 and 995–9.

Culliton BJ (1984) Medical education under fire. Science 226: 419–20.

Department of Health (1989) Working for Patients. London: HMSO.

Dewey J (1900) The School and Society. Chicago: University of Chicago Press.

Elston MA (1993) Women Doctors in a changing Profession: The Case in Britain. In E Riska, K Wegar (eds) Gender Work and Medicine: Women and the Medical Division of Labour. London: Sage, pp. 27–61.

Engel GL (1977) The need for a new medical model: a challenge for biomedicine. Science 196: 129–36.

Engelhardt JR (1977) Defining occupational therapy – the meaning of therapy and the virtues of occupation. American Journal of Occupational Therapy 31(10): 666–72.

Freidson E (1970) Profession of Medicine – A Study of the Sociology of Applied Knowledge. New York: Dodd, Mead & Company.

Fuller AR (1983) Synthesizing the everyday world. The Journal of Mind and Behaviour 4(3): 369–87.

Griffiths R (1988) Community Care: Agenda for Action. London: HMSO Publications.

Griffiths Report (1983) London: Department of Health and Social Security.

Ham C (1981) Policy-making in the National Health Service. Macmillan Journal of Medical Ethics 16: 178–84.

Hewa S, Hetheringon R (1990) Specialists Without Spirit: Crisis in the Nursing Profession.

Hugman R (1991) Power in Caring Professions. London: Macmillan.

Hunter DJ (1991) Managing medicine: a response to the 'crisis'. Social Science and Medicine 32: 441–8.

Illich ID (1972) Celebration of awareness: a call for institutional revolution. Harmondsworth: Penguin.

Innui TS, Carter WB (1985) Problems and Prospects for Health Service Research on Provider–Patient Communication. Medical Care 23(5): 521–38.

Jenkins MM (1994a) Occupational Therapy – Perspectives on the Effectiveness of Practice. Unpublished DPhil Thesis, Londonderry: University of Ulster, Magee College.

Jenkins MM (1994b) The changing ethos of health care professions. British Journal of Therapy and Rehabilitation 1(3/4).

Jenkins MM, Brotherton C (1995a) In search of a theoretical framework for practice, Part 1. British Journal of Occupational Therapy 58(7): 280–5.

Jenkins MM, Brotherton C (1995b) In search of a theoretical framework for practice, Part 2. British Journal of Occupational Therapy 58(8): 332–6.

Jenkins MM, Brotherton C (1995c) Implications of a theoretical framework for Practice. British Journal of Occupational Theory 58(9): 392–6.

Jenkins MM, Mallet J, O'Neill E, McFadden M, Baird H (1994) Insights into practice communication: an interactional approach. British Journal of Occupational Therapy 57(8): 297–302.

Katon W, Kleinman A (1981) Doctor–patient negotiation and other social science strategies in patient care. In Eisenbert L, Kleinman A (eds) The Relevance of Social Science for Medicine. Dordrecht and Boston: Reidel.

Kleinman A, Eisenberg L, Good B (1978) Culture, illness and care: clinical lessons from anthropologic and cross-cultural research. Annals of Internal Medicine 88: 251–8.

Lacrosse MB (1975) Non verbal behavioiur and perceived counsellor attractiveness and persuasiveness. Journal of Counselling Psychology 22: 563–6.

Larkin GU (1988) Medical dominance in Britain: image and historical reality. The Millbank Quarterly 66(2): 117–32.

Lasserman P, Velody I (1989) Max Weber's 'Science As A Vocation'. London: Unwin Hyman.

Lave J (1988) The Culture and Acquisition and the Practice of Understanding. Institute for Research on Learning, Report No IRL88-0007. Palo Alto CA: pp. 1–19.

Lave J, Wenger E (1989) Situated Learning: Legitimate Peripheral Participation. Institute for Research on Learning, Report No IRL89-0013m. Palo Alto CA: pp. 1–41.

Lazare A, Eissenthal S, Wasserman L (1975) The customer approach to patienthood: attending to patient requests in a walk-in clinic. Archives of General Psychiatry 32: 553–8.

Meyer A (1922) The philosophy of occupation therapy. Archives of Occupational Therapy 1(1): 1–10.

Mishler EG (1984) The Discourse of Medicine: Dialectics of Medical Interviews. Norwood NY: Ablex.

Mocellin G (1988) A perspective on the principles and practice of occupational therapy. British Journal of Occupational Therapy 51(1): 4–7.

Parsons T (1951) Social structure and dynamic process: the case of modern medical practice. In The Social System. New York: The Free Press, pp. 428–79.

Peloquin SM (1991) Occupational therapy service: individual and collective understanding of the founders – Part 2. American Journal of Occupational Therapy 45(8): 733–44.

Preston T (1982) From the editor. Biomedical Communication (November/December).

Popper KR (1965) Conjectures and Refutations: The Growth of Scientific Knowledge. New York: Harper & Row.

Roter DL, Hall JA, Katz NR (1988, Patient–physician communication: a descriptive summary of the literature. Patient Education and Counselling 12: 99–119.

Schön DA (1987) Educating the Reflective Practitioner. San Francisco and London: Jossey-Bass.

Slagle EC (1934) Occupational therapy – recent methods and advances in the United States. Occupational Therapy and Rehabilitation 13: 289–98.

Spiegel T (1973) Position paper, as a monitor, 4: 1, 7. Available through American Psychological Association, Washington DC.

Stewart M (1984) What is a successful doctor–patient interview? A study of interactions and outcomes. Social Science and Medicine 19(2): 167–75.

Stewart M, Roter D (1989) Communicating with Medical Patients. Newbury Park CA: Sage Publications.

Thorne B (1992) Carl Rogers. London: Sage Publications.

Vanier J (1992) The Challenge of L'Arche. London: Darton, Longman & Todd.

Wasserman RC, Inni TS (1983) Systematic analysis of clinician-patient interactions: a critique of recent approaches with suggestions for future research. Medical Care 21(3): 279–93.

Watzlawick P, Beavin J, Jackson DO (1967) Pragmatics of Human Communication. New York: Norton.

Weber M (1958) (translated by T Parsons) The Protestant Ethic and the Spirit of Capitalism. New York: Scribner.

Whitehead AN (1926) Science and The Modern World Cambridge: Cambridge University Press.

Wilding (1982) Professional Power and Social Welfare. London: Routledge & Kegan Paul.

Williams J (1993) What is a Profession? Experience versus Expertise. In Walmley J, Reynolds J, Shakespeare P and Woolfe R (eds) Health, Welfare and Practice. London: Sage Publications.

Windsor, S (1991) Professional Foul. The Observer Magazine, p. 5

World Book Encyclopedia (1977) Chicago: Field Enterprises Educational Corporation.

Yerxa EJ (1967) Authentic occupational therapy. American Journal of Occupational Therapy 1: 1–9.

Yerxa EJ (1980) Occupational therapy's role in creating a future climate of caring. American Journal of Occupational Therapy 34(8): 529–34.

Zimmerman T (1974) Is professionalization the answer to improving health care? Americal Journal of Occupational Therapy 28(8): 465–68.

Chapter 4
Influences that shape our reasoning

SUSAN RYAN

Introduction

Many influences affect and shape the way that occupational therapists reason. This chapter will highlight some significant ones while acknowledging that there are other subtle trends within each that will not be addressed. It will concentrate mainly on macro rather than micro perspectives, even though the latter are vital elements in this complex area of study.

The allied health professions, such as nursing, occupational therapy and physiotherapy, have adopted the title 'clinical reasoning' unquestioningly. The context and nature of practice for some of these groups is very different. Practice cannot be prescribed. What is suitable for one place cannot be suitable for another and what is necessary for one person is not for another. If this line of thought is pursued then it follows that general principles, processes, theories and frames of reference should govern a professional's thinking. These should form a background that can be used as required and can be enmeshed with the client's needs so that the uniqueness of situations can be maintained. This integration has been suggested by Schön (1983, 1987), by West (1989, 1990) and by Fish (1995). Thus, a health professional working with an individual or a family over an extended period of time, or a therapist designing an ongoing intervention programme for a service, is thinking and reasoning very differently from one who is assessing, diagnosing or evaluating a limited situation, however complex. So the context and the role of the professional must always be stated when interpreting reasoning. If the continuum of health care is viewed as an overall story, then reasoning in acute care is completely different from reasoning in community care, even by the same person.

Many professionals work with clients and their families in an ongoing way, sometimes over considerable periods of time. The reasoning and thinking that inform this sort of practice cannot follow the hypothetico-deductive method, which is the preferred method within medicine. Setting up theories and testing them formally would be too limiting for health professionals working with the many variables found in long-term care. Reasoning in extended interventions incorporates inductive and creative thought, periods of reflection, times of problem solving and periodic decision making. This produces a pattern of reasoning that will be described later.

Each healthcare profession has its own roots, values, beliefs and ways of working and thinking. In the literature these are referred to as its particular orientation or epistemology. This base affects what the profession looks at and thinks about and so the ways of reasoning and the emphases can be different despite the fact that each profession is working towards the same goal – that of the wellbeing of the patient or client. Members of the healthcare team come from these different backgrounds, some of which are more scientific in a medical sense, some more technical, others more holistic, others more academic, whereas others are more practical.

The nature of practice also changes with the context of practice and this is another dimension that affects reasoning. Until recently, most professionals did not engage in any form of interdisciplinary study, and some remain ignorant of each other's interpretations and orientations. In addition to having different professional backgrounds, each team member has a varying number of years of experience. Thus, clinical reasoning in a team is influenced by a multitude of factors and only recently has research begun into these differences (Living R, personal communication, May 1997).

This chapter will range in scope from the cognitive and mathematical sciences to the psychological and anthropological sciences. It will intimate how these major divisions have been affected by different Western philosophies through the ages and highlight the changes that are occurring presently within medical science. It will look at the start of clinical reasoning studies and travel through their historical development as they continue to evolve. The discussion will show how the epistemological stance taken, consciously or unconsciously, by educators who deliver professional courses can affect the way initial practice is thought about and carried out. The clinical behaviour of beginners is often modified later through exposure to other ways of working or through engaging in scholarship where other views of practice or realisations about practice alter perceptions and personal stance (Savin-Baden 1997). In occupational therapy practice, conceptual models are often used to guide practice. These form further frameworks that affect reasoning and must be taken into consideration.

An issue that is causing debate between people studying this subject, and that will be considered, is the way that clinical reasoning itself is interpreted. Publications that purport to be about the same area of study often appear to be quite different and unrelated. This causes confusion for those who are not conversant with the scope of this subject.

All these controversies form the intricate background to this chapter. These influences will be interwoven with the changing nature and focus of occupational therapy practice itself to help the reader appreciate how the various studies of clinical reasoning within occupational therapy have been influenced.

Views of clinical reasoning

The word 'clinical' is not exactly appropriate for occupational therapy as it has connotations with medicine. Reasoning studies in the discipline of medicine have traditionally focused on a condition rather than on a unique set of human circumstances although now, in many medical schools, this focus is changing. In fact, it was the medical profession that started the initial studies, in the early 1970s, of what is now universally called clinical or medical reasoning. The focus of these studies was on the physical signs and symptoms of disease, which were viewed in a diagnostic sense. The information was reasoned through systematically in a hypothetico-deductive way, which eventuated in a decision that could be acted upon.

This section describes three schools of thought that directed these early studies and looks at parallel work that was done on adult learning. It concludes by describing three different models of clinical reasoning that are appropriate for different types of clinical practice.

Schools of thought

The major differences in approaches to clinical reasoning stem from the orientation of the early studies, therefore it is necessary to understand these roots. Process studies and developmental studies were conducted on different professions with different epistemologies, at different stages in their career development, and in clinical areas where there were different focuses of intervention. However, all this work centred on the reasoning of the health professionals. They were seen as the ones making decisions, and the patient or client was not included in the process as, at that time, it was considered appropriate and professional for the health care worker to 'do to' the patient. More recent work is considering the interdependent process of 'working with' or 'doing with' the client.

In the early 1970s, medical educators first started studying clinical reasoning. In the previous decade there had been an explosion of medical and scientific knowledge. The more progressive educators realised that medical students needed to be inculcated with ways of thinking that would embrace a continuing input of knowledge throughout their working lives. They emphasised that there must be an understanding of the principles and processes of learning in the under-graduate curriculum, rather than pure content. The ways of thinking and reasoning that developed from methods of teaching and the qualities of the teachers were of considerable interest to these educators. Three schools of thought began to develop alongside each other, although this was not recognised until 1987 when a symposium on clinical reasoning was held (Norman and Patel 1987).

Two of the schools were more scientifically oriented; these were the cognitive science and decision analysis-schools. The third school examined clinical reasoning from a psychological perspective and studied the representation of problems in memory. Each group made a different contribution to the knowledge base and understanding of clinical reasoning. Each, in turn, was influenced by other events that were happening simultaneously in parallel fields of study.

The cognitive science school

Cognitive science, as its name implies, looks at the neural processes governing memory, storage and retrieval, and the underlying networks associated with these. In the early 1970s, interest was developing rapidly in computer technology and the knowledge base of cognitive science is intimately bound with artificial intelligence, expert systems and hypothetico-deductive reasoning. From continuing work in this field, computers are becoming increasingly sophisticated and will soon be able to think, in terms of offering choices. In medicine, a way of reasoning based on the cognitive science school of thought centres around the expert procedures used to diagnose and treat medical problems. This method is grounded in the concept of expert reasoning and shows how reasoning might be taught. Computer programmes have already been developed to guide the medical student and the physician through symptomatologies.

The decision-making school

This school of thought focuses on how doctors make judgements and decisions when making a diagnosis and determining a course of action. This approach recognises that humans are prone to biases and so normative models have been developed that prescribe optimum decision-making rules for specific clinical situations. These are data-based aids that look at medical data from a clinical perspective. Some are based on mathematical probability theories.

The concept learning school

This approach emerged from psychological research where the primary concern was understanding how concepts or categories of information are represented in the memory. In particular, this school of thought theorises that experienced practitioners conceptualise practice in very different ways from beginners. Each experience encountered contributes to a memory trace. So, with increasing exposure to similar experiences, an accumulation of traces occurs. These are then matched to other situations and the relationships between one incident and another are mentally compared.

Adult learning

The early studies of clinical reasoning, whatever perspective they took, tried to understand the mental processes that occurred during clinical practice. These processes were often compared with expert systems, which some termed 'the gold standard'. It was at this time, in the late 1970s and early 1980s, that work on adult learning (androgogy), experiential learning and reflection was being proposed by authors such as Knowles, Kolb, and Schön and Argyris. These concepts are all interconnected with ways of learning and ways of reasoning.

In this period, another study was being conducted by Dreyfus and Dreyfus (1980). Stuart Dreyfus was a mathematician and his brother, Hubert, was a philosopher. They recognised the work from artificial intelligence and the scientific schools of thought but wanted to emphasise that this cognitive way of thinking and working should be treated merely as a tool and should be governed by the thinker.

Dreyfus and Dreyfus (1980) acknowledged that any learning problem has several dimensions that need to be considered. They realised that the focus of reasoning is different at certain stages of a person's learning and exposure to experience. In their study, they looked at the processes that adult learners go through when they learn something new, and they tried to understand where the learners focus their thoughts. These adult learners came from varied backgrounds, including airline pilots, chess players, automobile drivers and adult learners of a second language. From this diverse group, Dreyfus and Dreyfus identified five stages of skill acquisition, each of which involves a different approach to reasoning, ranging from novice to expert.

As ways of reasoning were being studied, it became evident in all schools of thought that experts reason very differently from novices. For instance, the cognitive science school believed that the neural systems and networks alter and reconfigure as they take in increasing amounts of information. The concept learning school believed that individual memory traces become 'chunked' together so that an expert can deal with familiar situations rapidly. The expert is able to recognise patterns and groups whereas the novice has to work through all the different elements trying to make sense from them. Time is, therefore, of prime importance. It is a factor that should be examined critically in any methodology that is aiming to study clinical reasoning. Beginners do need much more time.

A different view of expert medical practice came from the Netherlands in the late 1980s. Boshuizen and Schmidt (1995) believed that expert doctors have developed 'illness scripts' in their thinking. These can be instantly accessed and used automatically. Active reasoning is only used when some presenting features are unusual or unknown.

Benner, who came from a nursing background and carried out research with the Dreyfus brothers, later applied the five stages of skill acquisition as a framework for the development of thinking and reasoning in nurses (Benner 1984). The stages are currently being used as a developmental framework for some occupational therapy schools and fieldwork curricula in the UK and the USA. To date, no one has questioned the suitability of this framework for occupational therapists and few have criticised its application for nurses.

Three models of reasoning

The three models of reasoning outlined here appear to simplify the reasoning process but it is, in fact, complex. Any model must take into account the professional focus, the situations and the abundance of data with which therapists reason, all of which necessitate an understanding of the reasoning professional's role within a particular context.

Linear model

The classical form of general reasoning was described by the education-alist John Dewey in the 1930s. He outlined a five-stage process that included discovery, formulation and a conclusion from which various inferences could be drawn. The five stages are:

- reflecting on ideas,
- forming hypotheses,
- evaluating these for truth,
- determining an action, and
- forming a proposition where a verbal statement is made from the chosen hypothesis (cited in Fleming 1988).

This model is broadly similar to the hypothetico-deductive reasoning used in early medical studies. Figure 4.1 illustrates an interpretation of this form of reasoning which is not based on hypotheses but on assumptions, yet it follows a similar deductive scheme.

This model is included as it illustrates features that are not included in Dewey's description, such as depth of understanding. There is also a dual finale where the consequences and implications of the chosen action are contemplated. Following this model, the reasoner reflects on conclusions previously reached. Both outlines include inductive thought, although it is positioned differently. In Dewey's model, induction and reflection happen at the beginning and the middle of the

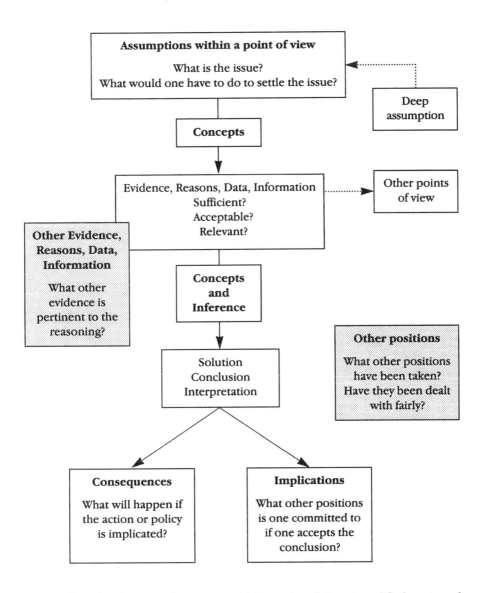

Figure 4.1: The elements of reasoning within a point of view. A modified version of schema originally devised by Ralph H Johnson; design and layout based on JA Blaire. Reprinted with permission from Paul R (1992) Centre for Critical Thinking, Sonana State University, California.

reasoning framework whereas this element flows throughout the second model, making thinking more critical.

Spiral model

A second and different model of reasoning was alluded to in the introduction to this chapter. Unlike the model just described, which occurs in more restricted circumstances, such as diagnosing, solving problems, or scrutinising points of view, this latter way of reasoning happens during prolonged periods of exposure when working with a client, for example, in rehabilitation settings of various kinds. Higgs and Jones (1995, p. 3, citing Cervero 1988 and Harris 1993) described: '. . . the thinking process directed towards enabling the clinician to take "wise" action, meaning taking the best judged action in a specific context.'

Figure 4.2 illustrates how this process is seen as an ever expanding spiral that interweaves all the elements of reasoning, thinking, and reflecting in both the client's and the clinician's frames of reference in an ongoing manner. The shape and ways of reasoning are entirely different from the hypothetico-deductive model, although this form of reasoning evidently occurs numerous times within the spiral and is subsumed within it. If this model is drawn more graphically, to include episodes of deductive reasoning, it may appear as a sausage-like chain.

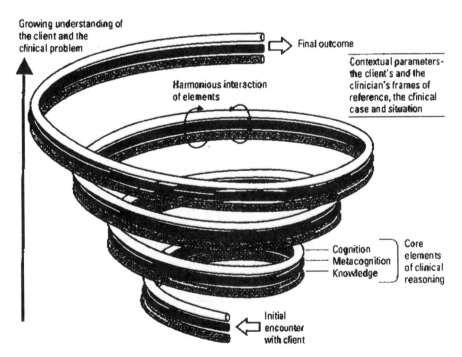

Figure 4.2: Clinical reasoning – overview. Reprinted with permission from Higgs J, Jones M (1995) Clinical Reasoning in the Health Sciences. Butterworth – Heinemann, Oxford.

Narrative model

Reasoning in practice can still be viewed in other ways. There is a distinction between complex practice and simple practice. According to Fortune and Ryan (1996) this differs for each therapist, as what is considered complex by one therapist may be simple for another. This perception of the complexity of practice is connected with the ability of the reasoner rather than depending on the length of the intervention or the amount of data available. Complex reasoning occurs when those involved in the intervention suffer multiple drawbacks and go through times of struggle, regression and reconfiguration before going forward. In the literature this is referred to as the 'swamp' of family life (Medhurst and Ryan 1996) or the messy low ground of practice (Schön 1983). Periods of reasoning can be reiterated to form a complex tangle rather than a symmetrical shape, as shown in Figure 4.3.

Reasoning can also be situated in the future as well as in the present. This conditional reasoning guides the shape of the immediate situation.

Influences on reasoning

So far, we have looked at models of clinical reasoning and how they are linked to particular ways of working or clinical contexts. This section considers more subtle influences on reasoning. These are discussed under two headings: educational influences and paradigms of knowledge. The section finishes with an overview of the history and professional paradigm of occupational therapy

Educational influences

Clinical reasoning is intimately bound with ways of learning. There are several educational influences that affect the novice practitioner's initial attempts at clinical reasoning, but much depends on the profession itself and its particular focus.

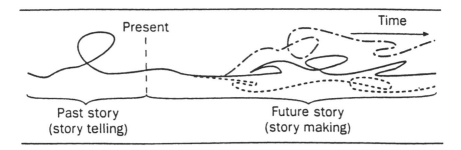

Figure 4.3: Diagrammatic representation of narrative time. Reprinted with permission from Medhurst A, Ryan S (1996) Clinical Reasoning in Local Authority Paediatric Occupational Therapy: Planning a major adaptation for the child with a degenerative condition. Part 1. The British Journal of Occupational Therapy. 59(5) 203–206.

The way a student learns to reason can be influenced by the philosophy of learning that is used throughout the course and, hence, the methods of teaching and learning that are employed and how these are mapped out for each succeeding year. At present, there is much debate in medicine and healthcare about the advantages or otherwise of problem-based learning (Savin-Baden 1997). Part of this debate is concerned with the way that basic sciences, theoretical subjects, practical experiences and research are integrated in the curriculum design. This includes the overall pattern of subjects within the curriculum and how they relate to assignments and work experience. These influences affect both the way that reasoning is approached and the quality of thinking. The learning and reasoning outcomes at every educational stage need to be identified and understood if better methods of educational delivery are to be devised.

In the UK, the national curricula in the health professions were deregulated in the 1980s. Schools became free to develop their own curricula and employ their preferred learning philosophies, as long as core elements were included. The thinking behind this academic freedom was that individual establishments could respond to local needs or develop unique centres.

In the same decade, there was a growing awareness of the healthcare consumer who was becoming increasingly knowledgeable about health, and demanding and critical of the services that were offered. Health care interventions supposedly became client-centred so that the individual's needs were considered in decision making or problem solving. This was a different orientation from profession-centred practice and, consequently, the practitioner's reasoning and ways of working had to alter to take this new perspective into account.

Conversely, in the new, market healthcare system, there was also a call from health service managers for standardisation of practice, leading to the erosion of the autonomy of the health care professions. On the one hand, innovation and individualisation were being encouraged whereas, on the other, ways of working and thinking were being regulated. Some health professionals found their performance being judged by behaviourial competencies.

Changes in consumer expectations and methods of health care influence the design of health curricula and the teaching methods used. This, in turn, influences how practitioners learn to reason and how they work after qualifying. Ways of teaching and working are also influenced by conceptualisations, in the wider society, of how the world can best be understood. Essentially, these represent different paradigms or worldviews. At the start of this chapter it was mentioned that health educationalists view their professions through particular epistemologies and paradigms. These paradigms affect the learning philosophies, the course designs and the way that learning experiences are handled.

Two important paradigms, the reductionist view of knowledge acquisition and the systems view, are described in the next section.

Paradigms of knowledge

For thousands of years, Western thinking has been influenced by the work of the early Greek philosophers such as Plato and Aristotle. The Western ideal of rationality and the pursuit of abstract knowledge can be traced back to ancient Greece. However, competing theorists and philosophers have always seen and attributed things very differently from each other, and so it is today, particularly with the study of clinical reasoning and thinking. In recent years, for example, De Bono (1991) directly challenged forms of reasoning which he referred to as the rock logic of Western thinking. He believed this way of reasoning is: 'based on rigid categories, absolutes, argument and adversarial point scoring'. Instead, he proposed the use of the water logic of perception.

Knowing that certain individuals or groups see things in other, and sometimes opposing, ways need not be seen as a threat. Interpretations of a word change through the centuries. What was meant by 'rational thought' in one period was different in another. One person may be rational when discussing a particular subject and irrational when discussing another. Learning and thinking about these different views can be exciting rather than threatening. When people feel easier with uncertainty and mystery, they can be freed from the constraining straightjacket formed in their minds that comes from thinking things are either right or wrong, done this way and not that way. Phenomena can be interpreted differently according to which view or perspective the individual chooses to take. Two ways of thinking are described here: scientific thinking and artistic thinking.

Reason has been at the heart of Western philosophy since its earliest recorded times. The early philosophers studied the natural world and sought to clarify, through discourse, listening, argument and questioning, their reasons for believing that phenomena work in particular ways.

It is possible to follow the history of reason through the ages of Antiquity, the Middle Ages, the Renaissance and the Baroque period to the age of Empiricism and Enlightenment. Reason has often been combined with the senses, compared with faith and seen as a primary source of knowledge, as well as being influenced by external and internal conditions.

The reasoning of the early philosophers was directed at natural phenomena and, as time progressed, thoughts moved towards discovering the laws behind and surrounding these. Moving through the centuries, it was in the seventeenth century in the Western world when scientific thought about the rules governing this physical world came to prominence. Creek (1997) described this as follows: 'As the scientific method achieves greater accuracy, reliability, objectivity and rationality, so we approach closer to the goal of absolute truth' (p. 50).

Reason has led to scientific progress. Through this way of thinking, great discoveries have been, and continue to be, made. Scientific thinking has dominated the medical profession for the greater part of this century and, inevitably, influenced the development of occupational therapy. Only in the 1970s and 1980s did an element of unease with the reductionist approach of science appear in the literature, particularly when it related to working with people.

Artistic thinking

In the past two decades, writers on reflective practice (Schön 1983 and Fish, Twinn and Purr 1990, 1991) have been promoting the art of practice along with science. Books by the neurologist Oliver Sachs (1985) started interweaving anthropological and thinking elements into a scientific and medical account. New qualitative research paradigms for the health sciences were proposed by Reason and Rowan (1981) among others. This new era coincided with the end of the modernist age and, in the late 1980s, the postmodernist era heralded new scientific visions. As Cornwell (1995) wrote:

> The wheel of science, however, continues to turn. Twentieth century discoveries of new phenomena at successive levels in matter, living organisms, and mind-brain relationships have led to a more dynamic, emergent, relational view of nature. There is a new emphasis on holism, on an appreciation of nature's complex combinations of structure and openness, law and chance, order and chaos, determinism and probability.

This new perspective is steadily emerging alongside the previous view of science. A view of humans as open systems has been embraced by some people and has altered their ways of working and thinking. Fish (1995) attempted to illustrate these two ways of working: the technical, rational approach based on scientific thinking and the practical, artistic approach based on a more dynamic, systems way of thinking (Table 4.1).

It has been argued that it is necessary to start learning in a technical rational way and then, with experience, progress to the other way of thinking and working. However, if the reflective and artistic methods of Schön (1987) or Eraut (1994), or the ideas of Barnitt (1990) on critical thinking, are incorporated into learning processes, then it is possible to understand and use procedural methods without becoming entrenched in, or smothered by, them. It seems entirely possible to start professional education from the artistic standpoint.

Table 4.1: Two models of professionalism

The technical rational view	The practical artistry view
Follows rules, laws, schedules; uses routines, prescriptions	Starts where rules fade; sees patterns, frameworks
Uses diagnosis/analysis to think about teaching	Uses interpretation and appreciation to think about teaching
Wants efficient systems	Wants creativity and room to be wrong
Sees knowledge as graspable, permanent	Sees knowledge as temporary, dynamic, problematic
Theory is applied to practice	Theory emerges from practice
Visible performance is central	There is more to it than the surface features
Setting out and testing for basic competences is vital	There is more to teaching than the sum of the parts
Technical expertise is all	Professional judgement counts
Sees professional activities as masterable	Sees mystery at the heart of the professional activities
Emphasises the known	Embraces uncertainty
Standards must be fixed; standards are measurable; standards must be controlled	That which is most easily fixed and measurable is also trivial – professionals should be trusted
Emphasises assessment, appraisal, inspection, accreditation	Emphasises investigation, reflection, deliberation
Change must be managed from outside	Professionals can develop from inside
Quality is really about quantity of that which is measurable	Quality comes from deepening insight to one's values, priorities, actions
Technical accountability	Professional answerability
This is training	This is education
Takes the instrumental view of learning	Sees education as intrinsically worth-while

Reprinted with permission
Source: Fish, D (1995) *Quality Mentoring for Student Teachers: A Principled Approach to Practice.* London: David Fulton

So far, we have been looking at the broader historical and epistemological context of clinical reasoning. The next section focuses on the profession of occupational therapy.

History and epistemology of occupational therapy

Each profession has its own roots from which came its basic truths. Where the underlying assumptions of the profession of occupational therapy fit in relation to health science, both at its beginnings and now, is an interesting question. Also of interest is the relationship between the development of the profession and the ways that practitioners think, reason and work.

Occupational therapy is not as old or well established as, for example, medicine. The origins of the profession centred on getting people to work in a balanced range of activities, but how and where this was done differed in different countries. In the USA, according to Mocellin (1992), people from the already-established disciplines of nursing, psychiatry, teaching, social work and architecture formed the original founding group of the profession. This professional mixture explains why the philosophical underpinnings of the new profession seem so coherent and holistic whereas the scientific knowledge base seems vague and widespread. The first group of occupational therapists to practise in the UK started working with mental health patients in Scotland in 1932. According to Jay, Mendez and Monteath (1992), these original therapists held art college diplomas. In Australia, in the 1920s, nurses worked with mentally ill patients using arts and crafts applied to everyday life. Then an Australian, Ethel May Francis, studied occupational therapy in Philadelphia, Pennsylvania. Subsequently, she completed a postgraduate scholarship at Dorset House, England before returning to Australia. She started a private practice in Melbourne and set the first professional standards in Australia (Anderson and Bell, 1988). One thing the profession had in common in all these countries was that it fell, in varying degrees, under the influence of the medical profession.

Herbert James Hall, a physician from Massachusetts, USA, in the early part of this century said that, 'Occupational therapy is the science of organised work for invalids' (quoted by Quiroga, 1995, p. 13). This brings in the word 'science' from the beginning of the profession. It can be argued that the profession's background is not truly scientific, although therapists working in the period from the 1950s to the 1980s in North America tried very hard to prove this was not the case. Therapists in this era followed the language, reasoning and research methodologies of scientific medicine, which were essentially quantitative and reductionistic. The degree of scientific credibility of occupational therapy practice still depends on the context of work; for example, some areas of treatment, such as sensory integration, fall in the realm of applied science.

However, Mocellin (1992) believed that the search for a scientific model to give professional legitimacy, both in academia and with the other health disciplines, has been a major professional concern and stumbling block over the last few decades.

The debate over whether or not occupational therapy can lay claim to being a scientific discipline continues to this day. Some therapists and educators adhere to a purely scientific view of working, allying themselves to the rationalist school of thought. Others embrace a more artistic way of thinking that combines scientific knowledge with an acknowledgement of human frailties and the foibles and biases of both therapist and client. These practitioners also acknowledge the complexities of the situations in which they find themselves working.

This detour into the profession's origins enables us to understand the different perspectives that have been taken in clinical reasoning studies in occupational therapy.

Reasoning in occupational therapy

One of the most significant influences that shapes the initial reasoning of an occupational therapy student or beginning practitioner is the occupational therapy process, consisting of initial interview, assessment, treatment and evaluation. This is often taught as a linear process that can be likened to the flow of reasoning in the hypothetico-deductive model, illustrated in Figure 4.1.

Usual practice, other than in acute care and very simple interventions, is not a linear process at all. Therapists working for long periods of time with people or programmes usually mix thinking, reflecting and reasoning in an ever widening spiral process, as depicted in Figure 4.2. As more knowledge is accumulated about the person, or the situation, or the problem, the consequent reasoning embraces all the new data. Complex situations make the reasoning process reverberate in tangled circles before it moves forward and upward in the spiral once more. Even the experienced therapist's professional knowledge may become deeper on reflection as further understanding and appreciation is achieved.

Clinical reasoning studies in occupational therapy

The earliest clinical reasoning study in occupational therapy was carried out by Rogers and Masagatani in the USA (1982). This study, which was akin to studies within the cognitive science or diagnostic schools of thought, examined the procedural thinking of therapists working with physically disabled patients during an initial assessment. This study led Rogers to compare medicine with occupational therapy (1982) and steered her thinking in a particular direction. In 1983, she was honoured for her professional contribution by being invited to deliver the Eleanor Clark Slagle lecture, looking at clinical reasoning: the ethics, science and art of occupational therapy. This paper heralded the acknowledgement of the art of practice and the start of a change of direction in thinking and reasoning.

In the period from 1983 to 1986, new theories of adult learning, models of reflection, and new research paradigms emerged in Europe and the USA. In 1986, Cheryl Mattingly, an anthropologist, undertook a major phenomenological study of occupational therapists working in a physical rehabilitation setting in Boston, Massachusetts. By commissioning a social scientist to carry out this study, the American Occupational Therapy Association and the American Research Foundation were making a statement about the position of the profession *vis à vis* medicine and science. Mattingly's PhD research was supervised by Professor Schön, so there is an obvious connection between new thinking in occupational therapy and the paradigm shift occurring in the wider society. Mattingly's work was a complete departure from all previous studies of clinical reasoning. She introduced narrative frameworks and considered the meanings that illness and disability have for clients and their families. She wrote of 'working with' the client and illustrated this with narratives. She used the holistic, dynamic, emergent view of practice that Cornwell (1995) had described in his book as the new scientific frontier.

Mattingly's work was the start of a series of narrative studies that illustrate the artistic side of occupational therapy practice. Peloquin (1989, 1993), in particular, showed how expert artistic practice, and the empathy and sensitivity that goes along with this way of working, can enrich a client's rehabilitation experience. Mattingly's work continues to influence many other occupational therapy theorists, including Kielhofner, who has incorporated these new constructs into his model of human occupation.

One year after Mattingly started her research she was joined by an occupational therapy educator, Maureen Hayes-Fleming. Coming from an educational perspective, and being an occupational therapist, Fleming made a more reductionist contribution to the study. However, reductionism was interpreted softly and terms were altered from the way they had been used in medical scientific studies. Fleming introduced the concept of the 'therapist with the three track mind' (1991) in which procedural, interactional and conditional reasoning are treated as separate functions. This work, taken in its entirety, is more allied to the ongoing spiral of Higgs and Jones (1995) than to the hypothetico-deductive pattern of reasoning.

Many professional benefits have been derived from Mattingly's and Fleming's work in clinical reasoning. The complicated nature of occupational therapy thinking has been acknowledged, at least within the profession, and, more importantly, the human relational side of practice has been legitimised. This contribution is enormous in that it gives more confidence and assurance to the way occupational therapists work, particularly the artistic rather than the scientific way of working.

Since the late 1980s, clinical reasoning studies have proliferated. Some have followed the scientific paradigm, others the artistic. Some have looked at the hypothetico-deductive way of reasoning, others have taken the inductive route. More recent studies, such as those published in the special edition on clinical reasoning of the *British Journal of Occupational Therapy* (volume 58, number 5, 1996), have gone beyond examining the processes of reasoning to suggest ways of using this new knowledge in practice (Fortune and Ryan 1996).

Models for practice

This chapter would be incomplete without an acknowledgement of the use of models of practice in occupational therapy. For various reasons, possibly prompted by uncertainty about the essence of occupational therapy practice, conceptual models have proliferated since the late 1960s. Their construction at that time was based on psychological work such as the study of thinking, like the concept learning school described earlier. However, these models are profession specific and are often generic rather than context specific. Consequently, some occupational therapists find themselves using models in settings, particularly medically oriented settings, where the complete model does not fit.

Following the framework of a model guides thinking and reasoning in certain ways. If a therapist has a repertoire of models at his or her disposal, and if they are used judiciously in particular settings, they can be very useful tools, particularly at the beginning stages of professional learning. The danger would be in adhering to one model without critical thought about its content. The end result of this way of thinking is confusion and even mindless practice. Rigidly following a model for practice can lead to clashes with other healthcare professionals, with resulting exclusion. This aspect of practice remains a challenge for the profession as clinical reasoning studies continue to probe and explore the way we think, reason, reflect and work.

References

Anderson B, Bell J (1988) Occupational Therapy: its Place in Australia's History. Sydney: NSW Association of Occupational Therapists.

Barnitt R (1990) Knowledge skills and attitudes; what happened to thinking? British Journal of Occupational Therapy 53(11): 450–6.

Benner P (1984) From Novice to Expert: Excellence and Power in Clinical Nursing Practice. London: Addison-Wesley.

Cervero R (1988) Effective Continuing Education for Professionals. San Francisco CA: Jossey-Bass.

Cornwell J (1995) Nature's Imagination: The Frontiers of Scientific Vision. Oxford: Oxford University Press.

Creek J (1997) . . . the truth is no longer out there. British Journal of Occupational Therapy 60(2): 50–2.

De Bono E (1991) I Am Right You Are Wrong. London: Penguin Books.

Dreyfus S, Dreyfus H (1980) Mind Over Machine. New York: Macmillan, The Free Press.

Eraut M (1994) Developing Professional Knowledge and Competence. London: Falmer Press

Fish D (1995) Quality Mentoring for Student Teachers. London: David Fulton.

Fish D, Twinn S, Purr B (1990) How to Enable Learning through Professional Practice. London: West London Institute.

Fish D, Twinn S, Purr B (1991) Promoting Reflection: Improving the Supervision of Practice in Health Visiting and Initial Teacher Training. London: West London Institute.

Fleming MH (1988) The Therapist with the Three Track Mind. Paper presented at a mini-course in clinical reasoning, the Annual Conference of the American Association of Occupational Therapists, Baltimore MD.

Fleming MH (1991) The therapist with the three-track mind. American Journal of Occupational Therapy. 45:1007–14.

Fortune T, Ryan S (1996) Applying clinical reasoning: a caseload management system for community occupational therapists. British Journal of Occupational Therapy 59(5): 207–11.

Harris I (1993) New expectations for professional competence. In Curry L, Wergin J et al. (eds) Educating Professionals: Responding to New Expectations for Competence and Accountability. San Francisco CA: Jossey-Bass.

Higgs J, Jones M (1995) Clinical Reasoning. In Higgs J and Jones M (eds) Clinical Reasoning in the Health Professions. Oxford: Butterworth-Heinemann.

Jay P, Mendez A, Monteath H (1992) The Diamond Jubilee of the Professional Association, 1932–92: an historical review. British Journal of Occupational Therapy 55(7): 252–6.

Kielhofner G (1985) Model of Human Occupation, theory and application. Philadelphia PA: FA Davis.

Medhurst A, Ryan S (1996) Clinical reasoning in Local Authority paediatric occupational therapy: planning a major adaptation for the child with a degenerative condition, Part 1. British Journal of Occupational Therapy 59(5): 203–6.

Mocellin G (1992) An overview of occupational therapy in the context of the American influence on the profession: Part 1. British Journal of Occupational Therapy 55(1): 7–12.

Norman G, Patel V (1987) Current models of clinical reasoning: implications for medical teaching. Proceedings of the Annual Conference of Research in Medical Education 26: 245–51.

Peloquin S (1989) The patient–therapist relationship in occupational therapy: understanding visions and images. American Journal of Occupational Therapy 44(1): 13–21.

Peloquin S (1993) The depersonalisation of patients: a profile gleaned from narratives. American Journal of Occupational Therapy 47(9): 830–7.

Quiroga V (1995) Occupational Therapy: The First Thirty Years – 1900 to 1930. The American Occupational Therapy. Bethseda: Association Inc.

Reason P, Rowan J (1981) Human Inquiry: a Sourcebook of New Paradigm Research. Chichester: John Wiley & Sons Ltd.

Rogers J (1982) Order and disorder in medicine and occupational therapy. American Journal of Occupational Therapy 36(1): 29–35.

Rogers J, Masagatani G (1982) Clinical reasoning of occupational therapists during the initial assessment of physically disabled patients. Journal of Occupational Therapy Research 2: 196–219.

Sachs O (1985) The Man who Mistook his Wife for a Hat. London: Duckworth.

Savin-Baden M (1997) Problem-Based Learning, Part 1: An innovation whose time has come. British Journal of Occupational Therapy 60(10): 447–50.

Schön D (1983) The Reflective Practitioner: How Professionals Think in Action. New York: Basic Books.

Schön D (1987) Educating the Reflective Practitioner: Towards a New Design for Teaching and Learning in the Professions. San Francisco CA: Jossey-Bass.

West W (1989) Perspectives on the past and future, Part 1. American Journal of Occupational Therapy 43(12): 787–90.

West W (1990) Perspectives on the past and future, Part 2. American Journal of Occupational Therapy. 44(1): 9–10.

Chapter 5
Reflective practice in health care

KIT SINCLAIR

Introduction

Reflection is the process of reviewing one's repertoire of experience and knowledge to invent novel approaches to complex problems. Reflection also provides data for self-evaluation and increases the learning from experience that is essential for competency (Saylor 1990).

Much literature on reflection comes from research related to education and nursing. Schön applied his research to professional practice, bringing reflection into the health care arena in the 1980s. Since then, reflection has been strongly in vogue. This chapter will review the role of reflection in daily life and explore the development of reflective skills as discussed in the literature. It will address ways of using reflection as a basis for becoming better practitioners and 'learners' as it is through learning from past experience and building on knowledge gained from these insights that we improve our practice.

What is reflection?

John Dewey describes reflection in 1933 in his seminal book entitled *How We Think*. He proposes that reflection is a specialised form of thinking which stems from doubt or perplexity in a directly experienced situation which, in turn, leads to purposeful inquiry and problem resolution. He states, 'the function of reflective thought is therefore to transform a situation in which there is experienced obscurity, doubt, conflict, disturbance of some sort, into a situation that is clear, coherent, settled, and harmonious' (p. 99). He suggests that reflective thinking moves us away from routine thinking and action which, he submits, is guided by tradition and external authority, toward reflective action, which requires active and careful consideration of beliefs and knowledge.

Reflection is usually based on socially constituted issues, that is, issues constructed symbolically by the mind through social interaction with others. These do not have the clear, well-defined solutions that may be found in mathematics or chemistry. Reflection is a natural process people engage in through their daily lives. People reflect on events, personal happenings, involvements, concerns or problem areas.

Process of reflection

Reflection in this context may consist of four parts. First, you do and experience. Second, you reflect on your experience – 'what does this mean to me?' 'what did I feel?' 'what did I learn?' and so on – so as to understand it in perspective. Third, you conceptualise the new insights, compare them with past experience, perhaps projecting to the future, and use them to shape a more adequate conception of the matter in question, a better theory of it. Fourth, you try out your revised theory and look for new feedback.

Self-reflection implies observing and putting interpretation on your own actions, for instance, considering your own intentions and motives as objects of thought. This process is not infallible as it involves your knowledge and perceptions of yourself, which may not be as others perceive you. The insights raise awareness to help integrate knowledge and gain control over your own thinking. Von Wright (1992) asserts that you cannot, however, control things of which you are not aware. The idea that learning involves a new way of seeing the world is possible only if we understand that the world can be seen in different ways.

Habit versus conscious reflection

Schön (1983) suggests that knowing in action is the sort of know-how we reveal in our intelligent action, which can be publicly observable physical performances like riding a bicycle or private operations like instant analysis of a balance sheet: knowing is in the action. This kind of action has been learned and habitualised and does not required further thinking or reflection unless something out of the ordinary intervenes in the normal operation – a car shoots out in front of the bike, or the balance sheet does not balance. Mezirow (1991) separates reflective action from non-reflective action. He describes habitual action (Schön's 'knowing in action'), thoughtful action and introspection as non-reflective. Thoughtful action suggests that learning remain within pre-existing meaning schemes and perspectives. Book learning might be placed in this category. Introspection lies in the affective domain and refers to thoughts about our feelings and ourselves. Mezirow suggests that it can involve recognition of feelings toward others but does not encompass the deeper level of why or how, the reassessment or testing of validity.

Reflective action, on the other hand, is the examination of what, how and why we perceive, think, feel, or act as we do.

Boud, Keogh and Walker (1985) contend that reflection is purposeful and intentional, multifaceted in the sense that thoughts as well as feelings are involved, and self-organised rather than externally driven. Reflection requires keen observation and reasoned analysis, as well as a view of knowledge as problematic and socially constructed rather than certain. The reference point for reflection is some event or concrete experience the learner is grappling with – the ill-structured problem.

To put this into the healthcare context, as the professional tries to make sense of a puzzling or interesting situation, he or she reflects on the pattern of assessment, decision-making, implementation or evaluation. For the expert practitioner, this reflection may be a deliberate attempt to prepare for a future clinical problem.

The role of metacognition in reflective practice

Metacognition seems to involve reflective understanding of the process under consideration and of the actor's role in it. Yussen (1985, p. 253) defines metacognition as that mental activity for which other mental states or processes become the object of reflection – knowing that you understand something. This knowing process and conception of understanding change and develop as people gain experience of knowing. People have to learn how to make use of this understanding in order to develop their conceptions further. Metacognition is self-regulated and purpose-driven behaviour entered into knowingly by the individual. The reflective practitioner monitors the effect of an action taken as well as the cognitive processes employed to make a decision (Spark-Langer and Colton 1991).

Some activities that might represent metacognitive activities include understanding what one needs to know, reflecting upon what one knows and does not know in order to reach the solution to a problem, using one's cognitive resources and time on the basis of a plan made in advance, monitoring progress, evaluating the outcomes of the plan and revising the plan based on reflection.

As stated above, reflection can be used to describe the cognitive processes that practitioners engage in when making decisions. They monitor the effects of actions as well as the cognitive processes employed in decision making. With each new client, the reflective practitioner attends to the problems, makes inferences or hypotheses and mentally checks these hypotheses by looking for relationships with prior experiences or other patients stored in memory. The practitioner then makes tentative decisions for action and thinks them through to identify possible consequences. Finally, the practitioner will choose and implement the course of action, evaluate the action and start over again.

The reflective practitioner

The novice does not have a repertoire of experience on which to base judgement. As suggested by Dreyfus and Dreyfus (1980), the novice practitioner develops through several stages of skill acquisition, starting from that of rule-follower able to recognise facts and features and make analogies but unable to use this information flexibly or creatively or to deal with unfamiliar situations.

Novices are less able to think a situation through quickly than are experts. This may be related to either the way in which information is stored in memory or the difficulty with decision making because of lack of automaticity. In the first explanation, information appears to be organised into a network of related facts, concepts, generalisations and experiences. The organised structures, called schemata, constitute our understanding of the world and allow individuals to store and access large bodies of information with enormous speed. Studies have shown that expert classroom teachers, for instance, have richly connected schemata to draw upon when making decisions. The second explanation concerning automaticity suggests that automatic scripts allow experts to handle common routines almost without conscious thought (Schön's knowing in action). Novices, however, must consciously think through every decision, thus inhibiting the mental flexibility required for expert practice. If experts do not have to spend time on routine, it can be deduced that they will then have more time to attend to those events that are more novel or important (Carter et al. 1988). These automatic scripts for action are probably stored as schemata. For example, an expert therapist is able to check accurately on the progress of an assigned remedial activity to promote elbow range while discussing in detail family issues affecting the client's ability to manage cooking and childcare.

Schemata do not automatically appear in a practitioner's mind. They are constructed though experience. This is a dual process of assimilation (fitting the new in with the old) and accommodation (changing the old mental organisation to incorporate the new) (Piaget 1978). This could imply that the broader the experience, the more schemata available, and we might wonder where that leaves the novice. Cognitive research quoted in educational literature suggests that we should teach the novice the schemata of the experts but does that subvert the lessons learned from constructivism? Do we not have to construct our own meaning and develop our own contextual knowledge and prior case-experience to develop our own wisdom of practice? For every unique situation we encounter, do we not have to draw on our own array of understanding and 'meaning' in order to name and frame the problem in our own perceived context?

Expert practitioners can model their skills and, through case discussion and demonstration of dealing with ill-structured problems, pass on some of their skills to less experienced therapists. The skills and knowledge gained must then be internalised and become part of the novice's repertoire in order to be useful.

Ill-structured problems, problem setting and framing

Argyris and Schön (1974) refer to technical rationality, which views intelligent practice as an application of knowledge to instrumental decisions and views professional practice as a process of problem solving. They suggest that this emphasis on problem solving ignores the 'problem setting' where we define the decisions to be made, goals and means of achievement. In professional practice, however, expert practitioners take an exploratory stance, reframing the problem and questioning its solvability, taking steps further than the traditional problem-solving process and involving a sense-making analysis.

Past experience is useful in framing problematic situations because the new situation can be seen as similar to past situations or combinations of past situations, or as different from past situations. Framing problems involves consideration of the uniqueness of the situation and people involved, social and professional norms of behaviour and expectations held by others. Problem setting is the process in which we name the things to which we will attend and the context in which we will attend to them (Schön 1983, p. 40). Problem framing is necessary to create a manageable situation out of a problematic one. One needs to step into the problematic situation, impose a frame on it and remain open to the situation's back-talk, thus framing new questions and new ends in view. The next step is to evaluate the problem to determine its solvability, the desirability of the solution and the consistency of the solution with the practitioner's own values and theories.

The process of problem framing and evaluating involves the practitioner in a 'sense making analysis of an ambiguous situation' (Kirby and Teddle 1989, p. 46). This requires an openness to novelty, complexity and ambiguity, which may then lead directly to reflective action. An individual who is threatened by ambiguity may perceive the situation as unsolvable and move away from it or perceive it unrealistically to make it fit expectations. It would appear that reflective practitioners have a high tolerance for ambiguity.

Theory adoption in practice

Parham (1986) argues that the reflective therapist uses theory as a key element in problem setting and problem solving in clinical practice. She believes that the development of sound reasoning in the professional therapist is dependent on providing experiences that promote reflection.

Kim (1993) states that theory choice is entrenched in reflections by practitioners. New theories and approaches are adopted, based on the practitioner's own view of the situation and on the meaning of the problems as understood by the practitioner from reflections on her own actions, reflections of the situation and reflections with the client. Reflection on practice and on reflection-in-action assist in theory development and testing in collaboration with the client.

Schön (1987) suggests that it is sometimes possible through the process of reflection on action to illuminate the knowledge used. He argues that practitioners may not be able to articulate the knowledge that they use and states explicitly that 'reflection in action is a process we can deliver without being able to say what we are doing'.

Skills required to be reflective

Atkins and Murphy (1993), in identifying key stages of reflection, indicate that self-awareness, an analysis of feelings and knowledge and the development of a new perspective are crucial to reflection. These include cognitive and affective skills – self-awareness, description, critical analysis, synthesis and evaluation. Their model is applied within the healthcare context.

Self-awareness involves an honest examination of how the situation has affected the individual and how the individual has affected the situation. Feelings often have a huge influence on our ability to reflect, that is, to interpret and respond to a situation. If a therapist is frustrated and angry about a doctor's unannounced discharge of a patient, reflective thought might be temporarily frozen by the intense feelings engendered. Until the therapist recognises and deals with these feelings it may be impossible to think of alternative approaches to assist the patient with the sudden change of circumstances.

Description of the event gives a comprehensive account of the situation, including what has happened and what circumstances have changed on the ward, for the patient and for the patient's family.

Critical analysis involves examining the components of the situation, identifying existing knowledge, challenging assumptions and imagining and exploring alternatives: why has the patient been discharged so suddenly, what are the consequences of discharge and what adjustments have to be made?

Synthesis is the integration of new knowledge with previous knowledge, perhaps as a creative way to solve problems and to predict likely consequences of actions. It involves thinking ahead to the issues that will confront the patient at home, considering methods of adjustment or alternative care and planning how to approach the patient with this knowledge.

Evaluation is defined as making judgements about the value of actions, and involves the use of criteria and standards. Even before the actual event of discharge, the therapist can apply known criteria and standards to judge the consequences of the action to be taken, and may ask 'Did I do the right thing? Was there something I missed?' Self-evaluation is necessary for professional autonomy. In order to be autonomous, therapists make judgements about standards of practice. These necessary self-evaluation skills depend on the ability to reflect on appropriate criteria and develop as therapists increase their clinical experience.

In order to assist the novice to develop expertise, practitioners need to review their approach to passing on their skills. Clinical teachers do not learn to teach solely by imitating experts or by guided remediation of past errors but are themselves researchers 'continually reframing their world of work in response to puzzling or surprising events of practice' (Russell 1985, p. 16). Russell and Spafford (1986) suggest that clinical educators can foster reflective practice if the education process is built on the teacher's own assumptions about and reactions to their own world of work. It is this ability, according to Russell and Spafford:

> to integrate research with practice in response to uncertainty and complexity that qualifies the practitioner for professional status. Reflection in action may provide the understanding of not only what expert practitioners do but also how they do it. This view assumes that professionals do utilise prevailing theory or theories of their field, but also draw on personal experiences and assumptions, and are willing to engage in on-the-spot research in formulating solutions to unique problems. (p. 19)

Jarvis (1992) contends that reflective practice cannot be defined because there is no theory of reflective practice. We can, however, describe what reflective practice might involve. Reflective practice may begin at the point where the taken-for-granted is questioned so that a potential learning situation is generated. Good reflective practitioners can also ask questions of themselves and about the taken-for-granted in their practice, which can lead to new learning. This is the beginning point where practitioners problematise their practice and learn afresh about both the knowledge and the skills and attitudes that their practice demands.

Jarvis (1992) further states that expertise is gained through successful practice. However, all actions are subject to habitualisation and run the danger of degenerating into routine. When professionals treat their patients as unique human beings, however, the danger of the practice becoming mindless decreases and the level of consciousness required by practice remains high. If an anticipated outcome has not materialised, the practitioner is forced to enquire why this is so and a new potential learning situation arises.

Reflective practice takes time, but today's practice often appears to be conducted in an ethos that encourages both the performance of correct procedures and efficiency. Efficiency sometimes seems to be equated with treating as many patients as possible within specified periods of time rather than taking time to consider all the possibilities of care. The structure of the profession seems to preclude reflection in practice. There is a definite need to teach managers and practitioners the efficacy of reflection in the long term as surely, by improving treatment, clients benefit and ultimately there is an improvement in service (and efficiency).

Practitioners need the confidence to take control of the situation and confidence in their ability to influence consequences. This personal causation requires that a practitioner be committed to the personal and professional values used in setting problems and taking action, and in accepting the consequences of those actions. Argyris and Schön (1974) find it to be implicit in the willingness to test assumptions openly. Without this commitment, innovative solutions are unlikely (Kirby and Teddle 1989).

Colton and Sparks-Langer (1993) suggest that the following aptitudes are necessary to reflective practice:

- Efficacy – practitioner's belief that they can have an impact on a client's situation and on the health care system.
- Flexibility – reflection requires taking another perspective, looking at the world through another's eyes to find new meanings and interpretations. It is necessary to be responsive to unexpected situations and on-the-spot adaptations and innovations as necessary.
- Social and moral responsibility – to care about others and contribute time to social causes, to participate actively in the development of their department and the health care system.
- Consciousness – like metacognition, the awareness of one's own thinking and decision making, the ability to explain to other professionals the reasoning behind a given action. The precision of language required to clarify one's own thinking or that of others clearly promotes deeper reflection and awareness of meaning.

Directions for self-development in reflection

In order to incorporate appropriate attitudes and skills as a basis for developing reflective practice it is useful for practitioners to consider various activities or approaches. These activities can be accomplished individually, with peers, or developed as departmental policy.

- Practitioners should attempt to foster growth in cognitive reflection through reflective journal writing, self-analysis of video/audiotapes, action research and analysis of selected treatments/interactions, coaching, assessment and discussion.

- Critical reflection can be promoted through close examination of cases that illustrate particular aspects of context, ethical/moral dilemmas and other elements of practice that will help the practitioners to develop a rich, flexible repertoire of ideas, attitudes and skills.
- Practitioners need opportunities to construct their own narrative, context-based meaning from information provided by research, theoretical frameworks or outside experts.
- Practitioners should examine critically the preconceptions of practice from various perspectives to allow for a flexible and thoughtful approach to practice.

Conclusion

A key to becoming a reflective practitioner is the motivation to grow and learn and the desire to be better than you are now.

In his book, *Educating the Reflective Practitioner,* Donald Schön states that the problems that professional practitioners face are rarely straightforward and clear. They are frequently complex and lack right answers. Often, they cannot be solved simply by the practitioner drawing on scientific or technical knowledge acquired at school. Skilful professional practice often depends less on factual knowledge or rigid

---

Table 5.1: Terminology

Reflection – a generic term for processes involved in exploring experience as a means of enhancing understanding (Boud et al. 1985).

Thoughtful action – non-reflective action.

Knowing in action – habitualised action that does not require conscious thinking, familiar routine.

Reflection in action – on-the-spot research in formulating solutions to unique problems, based on prevailing theory and drawing on personal experiences and assumptions (Kirby and Teddle 1989) without interrupting what is being done at the time.

Reflection on action – thinking back on what has been done in order to discover how knowing-in-action may have contributed to an unexpected outcome, how actions have altered the outcome, or whether to change practice because of the outcome (Crandall 1993).

Reflection on reflection in action – a metacognitive activity, reviewing the thinking process undertaken during activity which may have influenced change of method and outcome.

Metacognition – mental activity for which other mental states or processes become the object of reflection (Yussen 1985).

Expert practitioner – able to handle common routines almost without conscious thought and deal with ill-structured problems using own repertoire of knowledge and skills.

decision-making models than on the capacity to reflect before taking action in cases where established theories do not (directly) apply.

This is the 'art of practice'. It refers to practitioners unusually adept at handling situations of uncertainty, uniqueness and conflict.

The extra demands that practitioners face today require more than intuition, instinctive reaction or a prepackaged set of techniques or protocols. Therapists must reflect on what is taking place, correctly perceive what the options are in a critical and analytical way and make choices grounded in rational, conscious decision making to improve practice. As John Dewey wrote, 'the student needs to see on his own behalf and in his own way the relations between means and methods . . . and results . . . Nobody else can see for him, and he can't see just by being "told", although the right kind of telling may guide his seeing and thus help him see what he needs to see' (Schön 1987).

References

Argyris C, Schön D (1974) Theory in Practice: Increasing Professional Effectiveness. San Francisco CA: Jossey-Bass.

Atkins TW, Murphy K (1993) Reflection: a review of the literature. Journal of Advanced Nursing 18: 1188-92.

Boud D, Keogh R, Walker D (1985) Reflection: Turning Experience into Learning. London: Kogan Page.

Carter K, Cushing K, Sabers D, Stein P, Berliner D (1988) Expert-novice differences in perceiving and processing visual classroom information. Journal of Teacher Education. 39(3): 25-31.

Colton AB, Sparks-Langer GM (1993) A conceptual framework to guide the development of teacher reflection and decision making. Journal of Teacher Education 44(1): 45-54.

Crandall S (1993) How expert clinical educators teach what they know. Journal of Continuing Education in the Health Professions 13: 85-93

Dewey J (1933) How we Think: a Restatement of the Relation of Reflective Thinking to the Educative Process. Chicago IL: Henry Regnery Co.

Dreyfus S, Dreyfus H (1980) Mind Over Machine. New York: Macmillan, The Free Press.

Jarvis P (1992) Reflective practice and nursing nurse education today 12: 174-81.

Kim HS (1993) Putting theory into practice: problems and prospects. Journal of Advanced Nursing 18: 1632-9.

Kirby PC, Teddle C (1989) Development of the reflective teaching instrument. Journal of Research and Development in Education 22(4): 45-51.

Mezirow, J. (1991) A critical theory of adult learning and education. Nurse Educator 32(1): 3-24.

Parham LD (1986) Applying theory to practice. In Proceedings of the AOTA Conference on Education Target 2000 Rockville MD: AOTA (June 22-26): 119-22.

Piaget J (1978) The child's construction of reality. London: Routledge & Kegan Paul.

Russell TL (1985) Images of improving practice. Teacher Education Quarterly 12(3): 16-22.

Russell TL, Spafford C (1986) Teachers as Reflective Practitioners in Peer Clinical Supervision. Paper presented at the meeting of the American Educational Research Association, San Francisco CA, April, 1986.

Saylor CR (1990) Reflection and professional education: art, science and competency. Nurse Educator 15(2): 8-11.

Schön D (1983) The Reflective Practitioner: How Professionals think in Action. New York: Basic Books.

Schön D (1987) Educating the Reflective Practitioner. San Francisco CA: Jossey-Bass.

Spark-Langer GM, Colton AB (1991) Synthesis of research on teachers' reflective thinking. Educational Leadership (March): 37-44.

Von Wright J (1992) Reflections on reflection. Learning and Instruction 2: 59-68.

Yussen, Sr (1985) the role of metacognition in contemporary theories of cognitive development. In DL Forrest-Pressley, GE MacKinnon, GT Waller (eds) Metacognition, Cognition, and Human Performance, Volume 1. Theoretical Perspectives. New York: Academic Press.

Chapter 6
The virtuous therapist

ROSEMARY BARNITT

Introduction

Occupational therapists express concern that professional skills are not well defined and understood (Kelly 1995) at the same time as finding it difficult to offer simple explanations of what they do when questioned by patients, colleagues and employers. On the one hand, therapists have a desire to produce a list of practical skills that define the unique contribution of occupational therapy. On the other hand, therapists are more comfortable in describing professional activity as a process, with a key element being the values and beliefs of the profession. However, statements about professional values and beliefs tend to extol emotional, attitudinal and behavioural perfection on the part of the therapist, rather than the messy realities of practice. For example, in 1992 Young and Quinn expressed their therapy values as follows: 'We value a therapeutic relationship of mutual co-operation with the patient' and 'We acknowledge the subjective perspective of the client'. These are carried over into the Code of Ethics and Professional Conduct, published by the College of Occupational Therapists in 1995, which states that occupational therapists are 'strongly committed to client-centred practice and the involvement of the client as an equal partner'. Whether these values are desirable is not open to question, however, it might be realistic to suggest that therapists who strive to perform at such levels are saints, martyrs or fools. In 1993, Joyce wrote, in an opinion article, that occupational therapists were a 'steady, compliant, professional group', when what was needed in today's climate was a 'radical occupational therapist operating anarchically' and not a therapist blessed with 'conservatism and moderation'. This caused outrage to some members of the profession and led to heated debate in the letters column of the professional journal.

Why is it that occupational therapists are so concerned with being seen to be virtuous? Can criticism such as Joyce's be put down to envy or defensiveness on the part of other professionals who cannot match occupational therapy standards? Recent research has suggested that, instead of criticising therapists for 'being too nice', attention should be given to those therapists who struggle to live up to such ideals within 'rapid change in the health service' and 'autocratic management styles' that make working to high standards almost impossible, 'resulting in self-recrimination, frustration and disappointment' (Broom and Williams 1996). Which is the real therapist: the moderate with conservative values, practising virtuously against the odds, or the passive reactionary who wants a quiet life? During research into ethical dilemmas in therapy, a number of insights were gained into the thinking behind this issue of virtue. The following chapter explores some of the issues related to altruism and virtue in occupational therapy.

What is virtue?

Lafollette (1997) said that the notion of virtue had recently been 'reinjected into the public arena' but that for many people it remained a 'quaint' notion linked to chastity and humility: 'virtues possessed by the few – and usually the puritan'. Any understanding of virtue was linked to the social or political circumstances in which people lived. Related to these, Hill (1974) discussed the case of servility and whether this was a vice or a virtue. Hill argued that slaves were servile because this was a prudent way to behave to protect themselves and their families, whilst in less oppressive societies servility was seen as a vice. Hill also related virtue to the social or political influences on the role of women (which includes most therapists) in current society where, despite the rhetoric of equality, he suggested that women are still being taught to defer to men, as men's desires and interests are the more important. If this is still the case, it might help to explain the compliant relationship referred to by Joyce (1993), which is often between female therapists and male power figures in the health service.

A second aspect of virtue raised by Lafollette (1997) was that of the need for self-respect and of respect from others. Only if this condition was met could the individual, whether slave or woman, feel that he or she had rights and thus respect. However, attending to one's own needs and rights has also been viewed as synonymous with being an egoist, the person who is self-centred, unprincipled and unfeeling (Baier 1993). Baier went on to explain that, in ethics, egoism has several versions: first 'the promotion of one's own good beyond the morally permissible'; second, that while people justify their behaviour as generally 'good', deep down it is still aimed at 'own' good, and, third, that a higher level of morality can be achieved where 'own' good 'and the common good are both addressed'. The final two versions of egoism given by Baier were ethical egoism and rational egoism. In the former, the greatest good is achieved by adopting moral standards (values and beliefs) and, in the latter, by being able to reason about and justify behaviour (reasoning and reflection). For therapists, the moral standards and behaviour required from the professional are laid down in codes of ethics whereas the capacity to reason and reflect is a primary objective of professional education.

A further debate about virtue is to what extent it lies within the individual, is internalised; and the extent to which it is subject to environmental factors and to social and political pressure. In the former case, the therapist could be held responsible for the personal morality of their actions, whereas in the latter case the therapist could claim social pressure to behave in certain ways not always consistent with their personal values.

Thompson, Melia and Boyd (1994), whilst writing virtue off as having been 'suspect for some time' except for 'valedictory speeches' of praise, gave as the classical meaning of virtue, 'proficiency or excellence in performance'. The authors further divided virtue into 'egocentric' ethics, already mentioned, and 'altruistic' ethics in which the therapist 'will tend to sacrifice self-interest in the service of others, so that they may fulfil their potential' (p. 47). This debate about altruism, or the motivation to behave well, has been active since the ancient Greek philosophers, in particular Socrates, Plato and Aristotle. They were concerned with traits of character, and identified major and lesser virtues. Individuals were ranked in virtue from very virtuous to 'moral monsters' (Pence 1984). During the Enlightenment, Kant argued that virtuous people acted as purely rational agents, not influenced by ordinary desires but wanting to be viewed as good people. Rewards were gained from having done good to people who were suffering. Whether these 'moral saints' (Wolf 1982) with such character traits exist in therapy is interesting to consider.[1]

Virtue in occupational therapy

The claim might be made that the development of health professionals in the United Kingdom has partly been as a direct result of a lack of virtue in their predecessors. In nursing, this 'amoral' behaviour was epitomised in the description of Sairey Gamp, the nurse written about by Charles Dickens in Martin Chuzzlewit as a venal drunken woman. Descriptions of such 'camp followers', women who served as prostitutes while tending the sick and wounded, are found in accounts from the Napoleonic wars. The crusade that corrected these vices started when Florence Nightingale selected women with intelligence, education and strength of character to accompany her to nurse wounded soldiers in the Crimean War (Showalter 1987). Similarly, in physiotherapy, which emerged as a profession approximately 70 years after nursing, the techniques of massage were developed to counteract the 'sinful massage provided by the oldest profession'. The 'new' masseuses were committed to demonstrating their 'skill and propriety'. This was as a result of newspaper exposures in the 1890s of 'immoral massage establishments' (Robinson 1994). The point is seldom made that prostitutes and 'sinful masseuses' possibly provided a much-needed service before ladies of good works decided to clean them up. In occupational therapy, the link between questionable practices and the start of the profession is not as direct as for nursing and physiotherapy, however, its roots are clearly linked into the development of 'lay therapists' who provided domestic activities in the asylums of the late nineteenth century. Prior to this, in the majority of institutions, lunatics were considered as 'unfeeling brutes, ferocious animals that needed to be kept in check with chains, whips, straight waistcoats, barred windows and locked cells'.[2] This image was later modified to become 'objects of pity whose sanity might be restored by kindly care' (Showalter 1987). This 'kindly care' was seen to be the imposition, or reinstatement, of domestic routines and moral habit training. In the 1990s, over a hundred years later, occupational therapists still have a major belief that domestic routines are an important part of therapy and refer to the imposition of routines previously lacking as 'habilitation' and reinstatement as 'rehabilitation'.

With the development of the professions of nursing, physiotherapy and occupational therapy, the original individual goodwill or virtue that energised practice has slowly become institutionalised. This is seen through the introduction of registration schemes, criteria for professional suitability, control over education and the introduction of standards for behaviour and codes of ethics. While all of these systems can be seen to ensure safe practice and control over the selection, education and employment of therapists, this does not necessarily mean that therapists are virtuous; morally excellent people who use their powers to do good. In 1993, Joyce wrote that occupational therapists were 'sensible, thoughtful and caring people who put the patient first'. However, Joyce then went on to criticise therapists for being unimaginative and safe in their practices, and suggested that what was needed by patients was 'preparing people for the jobs market . . . and filling the vast vacuum of leisure time', which Joyce suggested was beyond the grasp and competence of an occupational therapist. This opinion caused consternation in the profession, with a principal concern being that 'they' did not understand the role of the occupational therapist. Overall, little mention was made of the fact that some therapists also have difficulty with this. It may not be sufficient for a therapist to behave impeccably and have high standards that demand recognition by others, at the same time as being unable to explain their role. A curious contradiction is evident here. On the one hand, therapists receive a full professional education and find it easy to obtain employment (apparently with a job description), and managers bewail the fact that staff are difficult to recruit, whilst, on the other hand, therapists complain that no one has defined the unique skills of occupational therapy and that colleagues do not understand the therapist's role.

Some of these issues currently facing occupational therapy are due to the relatively early stage of development of the profession. It could be argued that occupational therapists in the profession are currently at an adolescent stage where the search for meaning, and need for an internalised self-image and self-esteem, is pre-eminent and absorbs professional energy. This links to theories of moral development where a stage is reached at which people are concerned with whether they exist, and are dependent on the views of others to validate themselves and their practice (Rest and Narváez 1994). This also links with the third stage of moral development described by Kohlberg (1984) in which an individual is concerned with the morality of interpersonal concordance: be considerate, nice and kind and you will make friends. In other words, 'be virtuous; your behaviour will be beyond reproach, and you will gain respect'.

In a hard-driving and unpredictable world, it is perhaps not surprising that therapists' vulnerability is starting to show. The changing ethos of the health and social services has run counter to some therapists' beliefs. Virtue has been out of fashion (Lafollette 1997) and skills that are currently valued include the operation of power, manipulation, confrontation and aiming for personal rather than social benefit. These values are viewed by some therapists as neither particularly desirable nor respectable. However, there is some indication that social values are changing again (Heater 1990).

Therapists have to some extent been hampered in their professional growth and influence on health and social policies by the hierarchical patient referral arrangements that have existed for four decades between doctors and therapists. In the 1940s and 1950s, therapists worked on the basis of referrals from doctors. Some dissatisfaction with this was noted in the letters pages of the professional journal in the 1960s and 70s, with complaints about inappropriate referrals, lack of respect for the therapist's opinion and lack of understanding of what the therapist could offer. However, this was muted compared to physiotherapists who made formal complaints to the government of the day when, in 1962, a White Paper was published (Robinson 1994) which stated that 'Doctors should prescribe physiotherapy with the same precise therapeutic indications . . . as they have been prescribing drugs' (Robinson 1994). In 1995, similar differences in political strength have appeared between the two professions, with the College of Occupational Therapists accepting that supervising students should be done with goodwill as part of professional responsibility, while the Chartered Society of Physiotherapy has stated that without financial recognition students will not be supervised.

In view of these differences, occupational therapists could be viewed as either very wonderful people who happen to be around at a difficult political time or not very wonderful people who cling to outdated values and have not yet developed the skills of radical politics. Some of these issues came up during data collection for a series of studies being carried out into ethical dilemmas in therapy. The following sections deal with two studies. The first looked at the sources from which occupational therapy and physiotherapy students said they acquired moral values and the second at the values and beliefs of qualified therapists that were identified during a study of ethical reasoning.

Acquisition of moral values

In 1986, Rest wrote that because of their background 'people in the professions usually have at least average impulse control, self-discipline and self-regulation abilities, ego strength and social skills'. Rest explained the acquisition of these skills as being due to a number of factors: upbringing both at home and school, motivation, personality and opportunity. He specifically referred to growth in moral judgement as being linked to 'those who love to learn', 'the reflective' and those 'who take responsibility for themselves and their environs'. By 1994, he and Narváez were writing that educational opportunity influenced the development of moral judgement far more than age. However, moral judgement, defined as an individual being able to select which actions are right or wrong, is only one aspect of virtue. Rest and Narváez postulated three further aspects of moral behaviour or virtue: moral sensitivity, the ability to interpret a situation; moral motivation, the prioritising of values, and moral character, the courage and persistence to act morally.

Hunt (1993), when writing about nursing, said that people who chose to be nurses had well-developed moral values that led them to the profession. The implication of this would be that all that professional education could do would be to build on this pre-existing value system. To explore this further, a study was carried out with occupational therapy and physiotherapy students studying on four different undergraduate courses. A simple questionnaire was designed with one research question 'Where do you think your moral values come from?' This was followed by questions asking for biographical information, including age, sex and professional training. These questionnaires were given out as part of ethics or professional studies courses at the beginning of the second year of three-year programmes. The subjects were given a box to put a free response to the research question, and also a

Table 6.1: The effect of age and professional group on value sources

| Age group | 23– | | 24+ | |
Professional group	OT %	PT %	OT %	PT %
Source of values				
Parents/family	94	82	71	73
Reflection	42	46	74	41
Education	29	30	39	54
Peer group	52	55	38	42
Religion	16	32	18	13
Life experience	8	9	32	3
Total Ss	69	63	43	32

(Categories were not mutually exclusive)

checklist of possible sources of values, taken from the literature. The sample comprised 112 occupational therapy and 95 physiotherapy students. The following results (Table 6.1) show similarities and differences between the two professional groups and between younger and older students in their identification of moral sources.

As can be seen, the majority of students gave the influence of their parents and families as the source of their present values. Only the mature occupational therapy students had a second equivalent source, reflection. However, it should be noted that the majority of the older physiotherapy students were between the ages of 24 and 32, while the occupational therapy students were between 28 and 42. Also, more of the occupational therapists were married with families, 83 percent, compared with the physiotherapists, 32 percent.

Parents/family

Whereas most of the students in the younger age group referred to their parents and siblings as the major influence of their values, a number of the more mature students, particularly in occupational therapy, referred to the influence of their own family, husbands, wives, partners and children. The comments the students gave lead to two insights. The first, for the younger students, was the influence of changing patterns of socialisation once they left home. The second was the identification of positive and negative influences of families. This was found across both age and professional groups:

- 'I learnt my ethics/morals from my parents but since coming to college they have changed to become more similar to those of my peer group – I have become more of an individual but parental influence is still there.' (Age 19.)
- 'I don't share my parents' morals and ethics at all. I have developed

mine by rejecting their ideals and arriving at my own through life experience.' (Age 27.)
- 'My early moral beliefs were established by my parents and relatives. This gave me a foundation to build on through school, friends and later experiences. Religion also played a part. This is a very thorough and established way of getting moral standards.' (Age 20.)
- 'My parents were strict, straight-laced and unbending. My moral views were greatly influenced by these but as life progresses I am becoming more liberal and much less rigid.' (Age 40+)

Reflection

This category proved difficult to define but, as it was identified by over 40 percent of the sample, and in the case of the older occupational therapy students by 74 percent, it is clearly important. One persisting theme was that reflection was about 'working inside your head', 'working on the process' and 'active thinking to sort things out'. Reflection could be influenced by any of the other value sources but ownership of the fruits of reflection, usually the higher order values, was claimed by the student. This might be expected to be more common in the older students with more life experience, and this was the case for the occupational therapy students. However, the older physiotherapy students were no different in identifying this source from the younger students. Comments the students made included:

- 'I find that I self-examine and investigate. However, being with others through difficult or challenging experiences influences my values a lot.' (Age 41.)
- 'I am aware that a problem sits in my head and irritates me because I don't hold a view about it. It keeps popping out when it is triggered by a similar event. One day I'll sort it out.' (Age 22.)
- 'I examine my values when something goes wrong. I have to decide whether to adjust or stick up for something I have thought about a lot.' (Age 19.)
- I don't like uncertainty, I like to get things sorted. I like to think it through as soon as I have time, decide, box it, and put it in my mental filing cabinet. (Age 28.)

Education

The influence of education on acquisition of moral values was surprisingly low for all groups, with only the mature physiotherapists giving it as a significant factor. This is interesting because of the belief promoted by politicians and some educators that, where moral behaviour is felt to be deteriorating in a society, the solution is to teach moral values in educational programmes. If the results of the present study can be generalised, the most important sources of moral values are parents and family, and this held for all students. However, as with the comments about family influence on values, the reasons why education was an influence were not always obvious. The following quotations indicate why:

- 'Sometimes it was a particular teacher who I respected whose views I took on, at other times it was the subject, but I think people influence me more than book learning.' (Age 33.)
- 'You don't realise how much you find out at school, even when you are sitting there thinking this is a waste of time, because that's what you are supposed to say if you want to keep your friends.' (Age 19.)
- 'At school I mostly found out what people in authority said was right and wrong, it took me a while to work out they had no idea really, they just followed rigid rules.' (Age 20.)
- 'As a mature student I found a whole world of literature and ideas which I could take away and work on. You realise that, while other people's ideas matter, you have to sort it out for yourself.' (Age 27.)

Peer group

The influence of a peer group and friends has been identified in some of the above comments. This influence was more important to the younger rather than the older students. In particular, the increasing influence of new friends, when students left home to come to higher or tertiary education, was apparent:

- 'I thought my parents' values were right and was prepared to live life according to their rules. However people here [at university] seem quite happy living with a different set of rules and I am tempted to join them.' (Age 19.)
- 'Friends give opposing views and argue about morals. This helps me to formulate my own ideas.' (Age 19.)
- 'I listen to other people's views, decide which I can relate to best, and then take it on board.' (Age 20.)
- 'I learn most from friends I disagree with (racist comments or abuse of women).' (Age 29.)

Religion and life experience

Religion and life experience were fifth and sixth in importance for all the students. The two highest percentages were for religion, 32 percent of the younger physiotherapy students, and for life experiences, 32 percent of the older occupational therapy students. Although these sources were not given as frequently as others, those who held them felt strongly about these influences:

* 'I went to a convent where moral standards were drummed into you all the time. Although I am no longer a practising Catholic I find myself referring to them when faced with a difficult situation.' (Age 42.)
* 'I don't think a secular society can be a moral society, only God can do this, and reward us after this life.' (Age 20.)
* 'Things happen to you which make you reconsider your values. My dad died when I was fourteen, and since then I've realised that life is not fair.' (Age 19.)
* 'The best thing I ever did was set off travelling for two years. It made me question everything I had believed in and arrive at values which I would never have had if I'd stayed in this country.' (Age 30.)

A number of conclusions can be drawn from the results of this study on sources of values:

* Therapists in professional education identify parents and family most frequently as the most important influence on their moral development.
* Moral beliefs and principles are not necessarily fixed and change in the light of experience, in particular, contact with new social groups and challenging situations.
* Moral influences do not always operate 'to the good'. Some student therapists reported moral beliefs adopted as a consequence of rejecting those promoted by people close to them, in particular parents.

Ethical reasoning in therapy

To examine how the early intimations of virtue identified in the first study linked to behaviour in qualified therapists, a second study was carried out. Sixteen therapists, eight occupational therapists and eight physiotherapists, were asked to tell the story of an ethical dilemma which they had experienced at work. The resulting transcripts were subjected to a number of readings to analyse different features of ethical reasoning (Barnitt 1996). This led to a set of themes which fitted Lafollette's (1997) definition of virtue as self-respect and respect for others, and included altruism, social desirability, and social influence. It could be assumed that as a therapist the individual operated from the notion of altruism, from 'selfless disinterest', however, as a 'normal' human the individual might also hold selfish motives and have a need to be accepted by fellow professionals as well as clients, relatives or carers.

Young, in 1996, wrote a somewhat cynical but possibly realistic statement about the current state of morality in Western parliamentary life: 'It is not exactly an amoral world. It merely gives dissembling a higher priority than other worlds.'[3] In the present research, a tension was identified in the research stories between describing events that implied ownership of professional integrity, the selfless disinterest referred to above, events which indicated fallibility and 'loss of face' and normal human failings.

The following five sections give examples of areas of practice in therapy where the tension between behaving ethically and compromise were most evident.

Being seen to behave well

Baron (1988) described behaviour when dealing with difficult decisions as sometimes leading to a 'neglect of consequences of a choice for the feelings of others', and 'failure to recognise the conflict between self-interest and the interests of others'. Contrary to this, therapists in the research described situations where they indeed recognised these conflicts but, despite this, the need to retain a sense of worth and positive self-esteem proved too powerful. For example, narrators tended to allocate blame for 'wrong' actions to other participants, particularly other professionals, whilst allocating praise for 'right' actions to themselves. On occasion, this self-justification was quickly followed by insight into the device, for example, with regard to a potentially risky discharge from hospital: 'It's easier to say that the doctor should make the decision than accept that responsibility myself' and 'I am aware that I keep saying "I was unable to do" . . . while underneath I know that I'm relieved that I don't have to make that decision and I can put the responsibility and blame on someone else.'

Being responsible for morally right but unpopular actions

In a perfect world, a therapist would decide which decision or course of action was best, or most moral, and then implement it. In practice, therapists are confronted with many situations where this is not possible, for example, providing mobility or independence aids when there are resource shortages. Hard decisions have to made about who is most deserving, and the therapist has to cope with criticism or formal complaints from those who have gone without. During the interviews, the therapists were concerned to establish early on that, given the opportunity, they operated from 'right thoughts' and 'right actions'. However, all had found themselves in circumstances where they had had to either compromise these 'right actions' or become subject to unpopularity with the peer group or managers. An example of the former was where a therapist was asked to be signatory for treatment, usually electroconvulsive therapy (ECT) for a patient admitted compulsorily to hospital. If the therapist refused, usually because the patient's rejection of this treatment was known from previous admissions, the therapist could be subject to hostility from other staff who had to cope with the patient's difficult behaviour. There was also anxiety that refusing to agree to the treatment may have been the wrong decision and the patient would have recovered with it. However, there was then the anxiety that, if the therapist did agree, a patient once recovered might feel that their trust had been betrayed, and this lack of trust could negatively influence all other aspects of therapy.

Overall it appeared that, where the therapist respected the patients' wishes and believed the resulting actions were right, self-esteem was retained, but this could be at the cost of anxiety over the risks involved and loss of social support. An example of this was where elderly people, living in their own homes, were deteriorating physically or mentally and becoming a risk to themselves or others, but insisted on staying where they were. The therapist might come under pressure from neighbours, and staff in other services, to coerce or recommend that the elderly person be removed to residential care. If the therapist honoured the elderly person's wishes there was a risk that a major disaster might occur, whereas if the therapist honoured the neighbours' and colleagues' wishes, this could affect the sense of worth of both the client and the therapist.

In these difficult circumstances, therapists argued responsibility in two opposing directions. The first was doing what was right even if it led to unpopularity: 'my colleagues don't know how to size me up. They say that they can't work out how I make decisions because I don't describe it in the way they understand. It doesn't make me popular but I have learnt to live with that.' Second was compromising what was right, justified as 'if I make too many enemies amongst my colleagues they can influence what I will be able to do with other patients. I would gain the moral high ground on this occasion but the consequence could be long term.'

Inconsistency in applying professional values

A number of subjects extolled the virtue of one ethical principle at one point in the story and then justified the opposite argument later in the story. A classic example was the strongly argued case for patient/client autonomy as a general ethical principle that should be adopted when working with a patient, followed by an equally strong case for professional judgement overruling the patient's autonomy in the particular case being described. Justification for this could be that the patient was judged as 'incompetent', that the patient was not capable of giving 'informed consent' because the issues were complex and could not be fully understood, or that the patient or relatives would make requests which could not be met.

An example from occupational therapy concerned the therapist's sense of responsibility for influencing a patient's decision to 'keep her from harm' and 'I've had a lot of experience of this and have a pretty good idea of what she needs'. This particular patient had a mental health problem and wished to come off medication to see if she could manage without. Later in the interview the therapist said 'You should never say you have seen it all before as this is too risky; you should say to yourself "this is the one who may be different". Anyway you must respect this patient's wishes even if they conflict with yours.'

An example from physiotherapy concerned a patient who had a neurological condition and the therapist made a decision to override the patient's refusal of treatment on the grounds that the patient was not competent to refuse. Later in the interview she said 'You should always respect the patient's wishes in these circumstances. He's probably had physiotherapy before and knows what he is refusing. Our professional code states clearly that the patient is entitled to refuse.'

Consideration of choices

The therapists were asked in the interview if there was any other way of thinking about the ethical dilemma they had described. From the transcripts it was apparent that participants gave little consideration to alternative approaches. This could be for a number of reasons: that therapists did not consider choices much anyway, that choices had been considered initially but by the time the story was told to the researcher the therapist was happy to support the choice selected, or that the nature of the ethical dilemma was so stressful that the therapist has 'shut down' on their usual range of problem solving skills. There is some evidence that the level of emotion generated by an ethical dilemma reduces reflective decision making and leads to a limited range of solutions (Eraut 1985).

Helplessness

Concerns over the wish to behave well and yet not be in conflict with others, when added to uncertainty over which actions would lead to the best outcome, led the therapists to describe a sense of helplessness. This was raised in particular with regard to the high level of uncertainty confronting the therapist when deciding how to act to resolve an ethical dilemma. Feelings of anomie were present in a number of stories: 'I felt trapped in the events and there was nothing I could do to alter them. I'm normally quite positive and try to make the best of things but this time I felt useless.' 'You felt that the whole situation had spiralled out of control, there were so many people and levels involved. All you could do was stand on the sidelines feeling helpless.'

Other respondents expressed their anxiety through anger. This was particularly true when the events had not been resolved and dissonance was still present when the story was retold for this research. Statements about the need to find a solution and end the tension were present in most narratives. As some of the events spanned several months, these periods were remembered vividly as 'living through hell', 'didn't sleep for several nights' and 'I thought of nothing else morning, noon and night'.

In the face of the overwhelming demands therapists face when dealing with ethical dilemmas, is it reasonable to expect them to be 'virtuous'?

Discussion

A major theme emerging from the research was the expressed wish of participants to be, and to be seen to be, virtuous. This was explained in a number of ways: the need to retain personal integrity; to conform to the wishes of the professional group and wider social, legal and political groupings, and to avoid the pain of exposure for absent or wrong actions and resultant punishment, guilt and shame. Each of these reasons could be positive or negative, behaving well for the right reasons – selflessness – or for the wrong reasons – selfishness.

Gilbert (1989) described a pattern of beliefs held by people who want to be therapists. He saw them as basically desiring to co-operate with others because of the need for relationships that are central to personal meaning. This can be seen as positive where co-operation is possible but it also brings the risk of rejection and abandonment when conflict arises. Some of these fears emerged in the research described, with therapists, when faced with unresolvable dilemmas, becoming anxious about their competency or loss of respect and good relationships with colleagues. Gilbert also said that therapists were more likely to come from, or gravitate to, moralistic religions, and that by choosing a co-operative profession were likely to find themselves in conflict-ridden or moral dilemma-prone settings. He went on to say that co-operative therapists might come from families that placed a high value on duty but low value on affection. This would lead to them seeking work that gave opportunity for esteem and recognition and would be highly achievement oriented. These therapists would be looking for appreciation rather than dominance. This theme of the desire for recognition and appreciation of effort was found in the present research.

Kagan, in 1984, questioned the notion of virtue and said that altruism and virtue were human inventions, 'they are prepared to invent and believe in some ethical mission . . . humans want to believe there is a more or less virtuous outcome.' However, as humans do believe in virtue it cannot be ignored, and the therapists in this research had no difficulty in describing good behaviour and good outcomes. They also described a number of altruistic beliefs, such as the belief that therapists were there to help patients, that at times the patient's needs were super-ordinate to the therapist's and that, by behaving well, the therapist might have to accept blame for an unwelcome outcome. Gilbert (1989) wrote that therapists had a right to make provision for their own good, at the same time as doing good to, or avoiding harm to, others. Where both were possible, happiness ensued and the event was unlikely to be described as a moral dilemma. Where only one party had good done to them guilt might ensue if the therapist was the party who had benefited most; and anger and frustration would be encountered where neither party benefited, or both suffered. These latter cases were likely to be described as moral dilemmas.[4]

Rushton et al. (1986) found that altruistic motives increased with age while aggressive motives decreased, and that altruism was found more in women than in men. In the present research, some differences were found between younger and older subjects, however, as the majority of the sample was female no conclusions could be drawn about gender differences.

A number of subjects in the research referred negatively to their professional skills and personal competency when these were under threat during a dilemma. Beck (1967) referred to the 'deception of competency' where people deny their competency – 'am I good enough for this?' – or say they are no good because of a fear of being discovered as inadequate. Therapists described feelings of doubt about their professional skills when these did not lead to a 'successful' outcome: 'did I do the right thing?' 'could I have done more?' A number of the dilemmas made the participating therapists feel helpless and damaged their confidence. Tillich (1977) described this existential guilt as 'negative self-evaluation to live up to one's own potential, it is a kind of self-condemnation for lack of courage in life'. The therapists who made unpopular decisions and who carried out unpopular acts were more likely to describe anger and frustration rather than helplessness when telling the dilemma story, whereas those who went along with social pressure, the popular act, were more likely to describe feelings of helplessness when the decision ran counter to their values.

Are therapists aiming for virtue, to act honourably to the highest ethical standard for their patients in all situations, or are they aiming to attend to their own needs in the hope that both interests will be served? Ellard (1993) said that there is always a tension between the two and that health professionals have to learn to live with paradox. He quoted from Galen's *De Placitas* (quoted in Burns 1977), in which a distinction is made between medicine and one's motives for practising it. The only obligation on the physician was to be competent, whereas motives such as glory, money or philanthropy were all acceptable. Perhaps therapists have been excessively influenced by Christianity, particularly Calvinistic ideas of moral behaviour with the threat of punishment for poor attitudes and behaviour.[5] Such standards require constant renegotiation in the light of cultural, especially political, change in healthcare contexts. The notion that therapists wish to be virtuous and act to the highest moral good may just be a myth, widely promulgated in codes of practice because this is the 'flavour of the age'. It may be no accident that an increased interest in professional misconduct procedures, and standards and codes of practice, is happening at a time when it is increasingly difficult to 'behave well' because of rapid change in technology and resources. Certainly, the therapists in this research appear to have been healthily selfish in wanting to do good, if this were possible, but also wanting to retain face and self-esteem, keep out of trouble (on the whole) and not carry guilt or shame after the event. As one participant said, 'Ten years ago I was supposed to care for my patient, now I'm supposed to be efficient and work within resource restrictions. Does this mean that I should get a new set of morals, or are the old ones still supposed to work?'

In addition to personal virtue, the therapists were well aware that they were influenced by the social context in which they worked, in particular having to consider power relationships and how these influenced the course of the dilemmas.

Power and control

The British Medical Association Handbook, *Philosophy and Practice of Medical Ethics* (Rowe et al. 1988) starts with the statement: 'Doctors use technical skills and expertise which the untrained person does not have. Possessing these skills gives him great power over his patients who by the very fact of being a patient are dependent, ill, and vulnerable.' The same might be said to some extent of therapists, although the fact that therapists work in a number of settings where they are dependent on referrals from doctors does influence this. In the research the therapists expressed relief that doctors held power, and thus responsibility, but were equally frustrated by this. Examples of the former were where it was considered appropriate for a patient to be told she had terminal cancer 'the doctors should do it, we are not trained as physiotherapists to do it', and where patients had apparently factitious disorders 'it's the doctor's problem, I feel like going down to the surgery and dumping it on him'. Examples of the latter were when the therapist felt more competent to diagnose musculoskeletal injuries than a general practitioner, or where the therapist felt they knew the patient's wishes with regard to ECT better than the consultant.

Increasing powers were also seen to be held by patients and their relatives who were learning to demand rights to services and felt able to refuse treatment. Examples were given of relatives insisting that the patient had 'more' therapy despite the therapist having made a professional judgement that the patient could not benefit further, and patients refusing to go into hospital, or refusing to be discharged home. In these circumstances, the therapist's expertise was challenged and a number of the participants described the difficulty they had in coming to terms with this. It appeared that patients living at home or 'in the community' were considered more prone to making their own decisions and assuming a position of power than hospital patients. This may be because the sicker patients are in hospital and are less vigorous in voicing their demands, or because hospital patients lose control over aspects of their life following admission and feel helpless in the face of professionals.

A special case in power relationships found in the research was when the patient was 'incompetent' due to intellectual or emotional disabilities. This was particularly true for occupational therapists working in mental health settings. A number of the dilemmas described were about patients who were not expected to be able to make decisions and the therapist or others had to accept responsibility for making decisions on their behalf. An example related to resuscitation when the decision for or against was made by a doctor without consultation with the patient, relatives or other members of the multidisciplinary team.

A number of forms of power (Handy 1985) emerged in the dilemmas. First was expert power: who had the best skills? Expert power was claimed by all groups of players in this research. Families felt they knew what was best for a relative, in addition to medical, nursing and therapy claims of expertise. Occasionally, the patient claimed expertise: patients with mental health problems who 'knew' that electroconvulsive therapy would not help them, patients who 'knew' that particular aids and adaptations would allow them to live independently at home, and patients who self-diagnosed and requested therapy to ameliorate what they perceived to be the problem. Second, was position power, the status of each person in the dilemma with regard to each other. The dilemmas identified the traditional hospital hierarchical structure as still being strong, with consultant/junior doctor/nurse/therapist/relative/patient in descending order still providing a formidable control. When therapists reported that their 'views' were not respected, this was commonly with regard to medical colleagues or patients' relatives, but occasionally to members of health management teams. This leads to the third power base: resource power. Issues around resources were common in the dilemmas where control over budgets, staffing and equipment were frequently seen as a problem. The ability to work ethically and 'give of your best' was seen to be compromised by: too few or too short treatments, particularly in physiotherapy out-patient departments; limits to patients' independence at home due to financial controls on aids and adaptations, particularly for occupational therapists; the perceived malevolent influence of fundholding general practices restricting the services that could be provided, and the difficulty of providing services for elderly patients particularly in residential care. The final form of power found in this research was 'legal' power. A feature of the health service reforms has been the notion of contracting and rights. Some patients and their relatives described in the dilemmas believed that they had entitlement to services, and that this was supported by documents such as The Patient's Charter (Department of Health 1991). Therapists reported conflict about these rights as being a major feature of some dilemmas: 'she said she would lodge a formal complaint with my manager', 'he said he would seek legal advice, or go to his councillor if the adaptations were not provided.'

Gilbert (1989) wrote that 'we would be advised not to ignore the role of status threat, need for power and hostility proneness. These may have a greater bearing on actual behaviour even in the presence of articulated moral belief.' In a number of the dilemmas, the therapists became more concerned with their role and status in the department than with the best interest of the patient: 'what will the team think if . . .?' 'I have to go on working with them long after the patient has gone.' Some therapists expressed powerlessness as a result of events in the dilemma: 'at the end of it I decided that as I had no power, what happened had nothing to do with me. I can't stop things or make it happen. I can't be held responsible'. Cooper (1986) wrote that some problems arise because the participants in the dilemma hold different purposes, and therefore do not value each others' perspective. Co-operation, which is an espoused therapeutic value, if not always practised, can work only if dominant hierarchies are reduced (Chance 1980). While staff are caught into 'defensive spacing and the need to be constantly self-protective', which is true within many health service hierarchies, individuals are not free to use their creative reasoning abilities or 'operate in the higher moral realms' (Gilbert 1989). Despite some of these pessimistic comments, in recent years therapists have begun to challenge medical dominance, although this has been a 'diffuse and muted development' (Watkins 1987) and means that therapists have to be willing to accept the responsibility that accompanies power.

Conclusion

Therapists have been accused of being 'too nice', and steady, unimaginative, and compliant in their practices (Joyce 1993). This fits with the notion of virtue defined by Lafollette (1997) as chastity or humility, a moral puritan. Whether therapists are altruists and 'sacrifice self-interest in the services of others' (Thompson, Melia and Boyd 1994), or whether therapists are 'self-centred, unprincipled and unfeeling' (Baier 1993) has been the subject of this chapter. From the research reported, it can be seen that therapists struggle with the tension between doing good to others and doing good to themselves, and are not all the well-behaved, conformist individuals described by Joyce. A further struggle was found between the therapist and the context of the dilemmas that they faced. Therapists were not free to make independent, personally virtuous decisions, as on many occasions they had to take into account other participants' wishes, in particular those of people who were more senior in the health hierarchy and patients, relatives and carers who claim increasing rights over services. Student therapists reported that family and parents were the most frequent influence over their acquisition of moral beliefs and standards, however, these beliefs and standards were subject to change as a result of experience, leaving home and a new social group for younger students, and travel and reflection for older students. The capacity to develop ethical reasoning further, in conjunction with experience, should be built on during professional development. The influence of explicit statements about values and beliefs of the profession leading to virtuous behaviour and laid down in professional codes of ethics did not appear to have much influence, as few of the therapists had read or used them.

The conclusion is drawn that therapists make claims to be virtuous, but in practice describe the same healthy selfishness of any group or individual who want to survive in health care. Whether they can become the radical anarchists suggested by Joyce (1993) will have to wait until the profession has matured further.

Notes

This chapter was read and commented on by a professional colleague, Ms Jani Grisbrooke, whose knowledge of historical and current socio-political systems and literary sources I value. A number of points made in the article were developed or balanced by her suggestions. Key ones are given below.

1   The case given is founded in psychology, the study of the personal virtue vested in individuals. There is also the parallel aspect of civic virtue, a social and political identity, a loyalty to mankind as a whole. Marcus Aurelius (quoted in Heater 1990, p. 12) described the movement from the individual with the common capacity for intelligence and reason leading towards law in common, citizenship and, ultimately, the universe. A number of classical and later writers (Heater 1990, p. 13) have identified the tensions apparent between temporal civic virtue and spiritual personal virtue. In these circumstances where should loyalty lie, to the profession of occupational

therapy, the state that operates the health service in which occupational therapists practice, or to the self? (Heater 1990.)

2   A further link might be proposed between lack of virtue and madness itself. For example, in *Jane Eyre*, Rochester's mad wife was described as 'intemperate and unchaste'. Consideration may also be given to where virtue resides: is it in the carer who attempts to rescue the mad person, in the 'mad' person who may be expressing sanity in a 'mad' world, in the mad person as the one who makes the most effort by recovering, or in the carer who attempts rescue even though his or her own virtue may be contaminated?

3   The amoral or unethical politician is not particular to the time, but has been well documented in both fictional and non-fictional writing. For example, Shakespeare referred to politicians, in *King Lear*: 'Get thee glass eyes, and like a scurvy politician seem to see the things thou doesn't.' Dean Acheson, an American politician, when reporting on the Cuban missile crisis in 1967 recorded 'the irrelevance of supposed moral considerations . . . moral talk did not bear on the problem'. The supposedly classic example of an unethical politician is Machiavelli, who wrote about the 'necessary immorality' of politics on the basis that a good man would come to ruin when surrounded by those who are not so good. More recently Sartre, in a play called *Dirty Hands*, expressed the view that it was impossible to be a politician unless the person was willing 'to violate important moral standards which prevailed outside politics' (Coady 1993).

4   Another view of virtue which might be of relevance here is that it may all be a matter of genetic inheritance, following on the evolutionary theories of Charles Darwin. One-hundred-and-thirty years later, Richard Dawkins wrote a book linked to evolutionary theory entitled *The Selfish Gene* (1989). As the book is an exploration of selfishness and altruism, it could as well have been entitled *The Virtuous Gene*.

5   This comment is limited to one narrow band of Christian development and, whereas Calvin and his followers may have influenced a range of Christians in Northern Europe during the sixteenth and seventeenth centuries, in the United Kingdom in the late twentieth century such fundamentalist views are possibly restricted to parts of Scotland, Wales and Northern England. Other explanations are therefore needed to explore why therapists want to behave well. In the nineteenth and early twentieth centuries, getting into the 'caring' professions was just about acceptable for women who aspired to work, and gave them some measure of freedom in getting out of the parental home prior to, or instead of, marriage. The effect of the development of the British Empire on women's independence should also be considered. This is well described in Trollope (1983). The demands of the Empire for nurses, teachers and missionaries overseas, and the special status of daughters 'released' to nurse

soldiers fighting for such a noble cause, led to escape and the 'possibility of passion' (p. 147) at the same time as upholding British virtues. For the early years of occupational therapy, the 1940s through to the 1970s, recruits were predominantly from professional middle-class females with a tradition of public service (Hugman 1991).

References

Baier K (1993) Egoism. In Singer P (ed.) A Companion to Ethics. Oxford: Blackwell, pp 197-204.

Barnitt RE (1996) An Investigation of Ethical Dilemmas in Occupational Therapy and Physiotherapy. Unpublished PhD thesis, University of London.

Baron J (1988) Thinking and Deciding. Cambridge: Cambridge University Press.

Beck AT (1967) Depression: Clinical, Experimental and Theoretical Aspects. New York: Harper & Row.

Broom JP, Williams J (1996) Occupational stress and neurological rehabilitation. Physiotherapy 82(11): 606-14.

Burns CR (ed.) (1977) Legacies in Law and Medicine. New York: Science History Publications.

Chance M (1980) An ethnological assessment of emotion. In R Plutchik and H Kellerman (eds) Emotion: Theory, Research and Experience. Volume 1. New York: Academic Press.

Coady CAJ (1993) Politics and the problem of dirty hands. In Singer P (ed.) A Companion to Ethics. Oxford: Blackwell, pp 373-83.

College of Occupational Therapists (1995) Code of Ethics and Professional Conduct for Occupational Therapists. London: Ethics Committee, College of Occupational Therapists.

Cooper C (1986) Job distress: recent research and the emerging role of the clinical occupational psychologist. Bulletin of the British Psychological Society 39: 325-31.

Dawkins R (1989) The Selfish Gene. 3 edn. Oxford: Oxford University Press.

Department of Health (1991) The Patient's Charter. London: Department of Health, HMSO.

Ellard J (1993) Medical ethics – fact or fiction? The Medical Journal of Australia 158: 460-4.

Eraut M (1985) Knowledge creation and knowledge use in professional context. Studies in Higher Education 10(2): 117-33.

Gilbert P (1989) Human Nature and Suffering. Hove and London: Lawrence Erlbaum Associates, pp 206-9, 237-9, 247-51.

Handy C (1985) Understanding Organisations. 3 edn. Harmondsworth: Penguin Books.

Heater D (1990) Citizenship: The Civic Ideal in World History, Politics and Education. London: Longman.

Hill TE (1974) Servility and self-respect. The Monist 57: 1.

Hugman R (1991) Power in Caring Professions. Basingstoke: Macmillan.

Hunt G (1993) Right from wrong. Nursing Times 89(25): 22.

Joyce L (1993) Occupational therapy: a cause without a rebel. British Journal of Occupational Therapy 56(12): 447.

Kagan J (1984) The Nature of the Child. New York: Basic Books.

Kelly G (1995) Rights, ethics and the spirit of occupation. British Journal of Occupational Therapy 58(2): 77.

Kohlberg L (1984) The Psychology of Moral Development (Vol 2). San Francisco CA: Harper & Row.

Lafollette H (ed.) (1997) Ethics in Practice: An Anthology. Cambridge MA: Blackwell Philosophy Anthologies, p. 254.

Machiavelli N (1532) The Prince. In Bandarella P, Musa M (1979) The Portable Machiavelli. Oxford: Oxford University Press.

Pence G (1984) Recent work on virtues. American Philosophical Quarterly 21: 281-7.

Rest JR (1986) Moral Development: Advances in Research and Theory. New York: Praeger Press, pp. 18-23.

Rest JR, Narváez D (eds) (1994) Moral Development in the Professions: Psychology and Applied Ethics. Hillsdale NJ: Lawrence Erlbaum Associates.

Robinson P (1994) Objectives, ethics and etiquette. Physiotherapy January 80: 8A-10A.

Rowe AJ, Fortes-Mayer KD, Horner JS, Macara AW, McKechnie S and Wilks M (1988) Philosophy and Practice of Medical Ethics. London: British Medical Association.

Rushton JP, Fulkrer DW, Neale MC, Nias DKB, Eysenck HJ (1986) Altruism and aggression: the heritability of individual differences. Journal of Personality and Social Psychology 50: 1192-8.

Showalter E (1987) The Female Malady: Women, Madness and English Culture 1830–80. London: Virago Press, p. 8.

Thompson IE, Melia KM, Boyd KM (1994) Nursing Ethics. Edinburgh: Churchill Livingstone, pp 46-7.

Tillich P (1977) The Courage To Be. London: Fountain Paperbacks.

Trollope J (1983) Britannia's Daughters: Women of the British Empire. London: Pimlico.

Watkins S (1987) Medicine and Labour: The Politics of a Profession. London: Lawrence & Wishart.

Wolf S (1982) Moral saints. Journal of Philosophy 79: 419-39.

Young H (1996) Parliamentary morality. Guardian, 17 February, p. 21.

Young ME, Quinn E (1992) Theories and Principles of Occupational Therapy. Edinburgh: Churchill Livingstone, p. 62.

Chapter 7
'You will measure outcomes'

PENNY SPREADBURY

Introduction

It is important for policy makers and managers of health services to ensure that any investment in health services results in an improved outcome for the population as a whole. In order to achieve this, they need outcome information that will enable them to obtain appropriate, high-quality and cost-effective services and to be certain that service users receive high-quality care on an individual basis.

At the individual practitioner level, a high-quality service can be maintained by means of involvement in activities such as clinical audit and the day-to-day use of evidence-based practice (see Figure 7.1). Burck (1978) makes a plea for all counselling, guidance and human services to demonstrate accountability through evaluation of their practice. Ellis (1988) asserts that the caring professions, like all public services, should be accountable for what they do. He finds that the supporting arguments for applying quality assurance within health services are economic, political and professional.

Background

Before starting to discuss quality initiatives, such as outcome measurement, it may be useful to recognise the economic and political pressures behind the so-called drive for improvements in the National Health Service (NHS) and acknowledge the unique problems in defining and measuring outcomes in the context of healthcare. The reasons for the recent NHS reforms and for rising patient expectations are, if we are to believe the Government, the economic decline of the 1970s followed by recovery and low levels of growth during the 1980s added to demographic pressures. The right-wing political philosophy of this period saw market forces as being the most efficient allocation mechanism for scarce

99

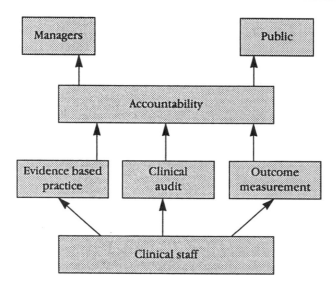

Figure 7.1: Quality assurance.

resources. The UK spends less per capita on health than many other comparable countries. For example, in 1987 we fell behind the USA, Sweden, Canada and the Netherlands. The apparently infinite need for spending on health does not match the finite resources available.

For the present debate on health outcomes we can thank Griffiths (1983) who placed quality firmly on the NHS agenda. He highlighted, in his report on care in the community, the problems of:

* a lack of continuous evaluation of performance against criteria
* little measure of health output
* little clinical and economic evaluation of practices
* no assessment of effectiveness in relation to the needs and expectations of people served.

The response to this report within the NHS, at the time of the newly implemented general management, was to appoint quality assurance officers, usually from a nursing background. Koch (1991) believes that this strategy had shortcomings because it moved quality off the personal agendas of general managers and failed to address the obvious cultural changes needed in order for the health services to enter an age of measurement of activity.

In order to allocate resources fairly, and in a way that makes economic sense, costs and benefits must be linked, ideally in a way that all can understand. Health service consumers should also understand the basis on which resources are allocated, as they pay for all health care, either indirectly through taxes, directly over the counter or via private insurance. In the quasi-market economy, provider units must provide what the customer wants or go out of business. Doctors, although often privately contracted, are agents for the customer (patient) and in many respects the patient's employee. The patient, in effect, buys in an expert agent to help him access the right health care for his needs. For many people, this not a situation they are able to use to their advantage since choice can be a responsibility that they do not want or with which they are unable to deal.

The reforms of the NHS during the late 1980s and early 1990s have encouraged purchasers to improve the efficiency and effectiveness of health care and this, in turn, has led to a recognition of the value of outcome assessment as a clinical and managerial tool. Purchasers acknowledge the need for more information on outcomes and, in a survey conducted by the UK Clearing House on Health Outcomes in 1993, purchasers indicated that they wanted advice on such issues as how to compare the performance of local providers and how to measure long-term outcomes. An increased interest from policy makers and managers in accountability has been mirrored by clinical staff realising the need to demonstrate the effectiveness of their interventions.

When examining the quality of a health service, it has been proposed that questions should be asked about its:

effectiveness
- Does the intervention meet the set objectives?
  Does the intervention match the outcome?
  Should the intervention take place or not?
  Who is setting the objectives?
  What decisions underpin service delivery?

efficiency
- Is the intervention achieved by optimum use of resources?

equality
- Is access to, and delivery of , health care equal across geographical location, age, sex, ethnicity and class?

- Is the provision and delivery of health care interventions sensitive to the complexity of individual needs, including dignity? (Strong and Robinson 1988)

Recent legislation, incorporating various Government White Papers, has reinforced the importance of improved quality and the internal market has brought quality initiatives, such as standard setting and clinic audit, to the foreground but it is not clear the extent to which these four issues have been incorporated into quality assurance initiatives. Many ideas and procedures seem to have been taken directly from industry without recognition that there are fundamental differences between the market for motor cars and the market for health services.

The first section of this chapter will discuss the tools that are used by managers to demonstrate the effectiveness of their services and show how they contribute to the maintenance of high quality healthcare. The next section considers what is meant by health outcomes and looks at the difficulty of setting and measuring outcomes in occupational therapy. This is illustrated by four case examples. The final section discusses the differences between therapy outcomes and individualised outcomes, arguing that occupational therapists should use the latter.

Ensuring quality

At the start of the 1990s, health service managers had three tools with which to implement the Government's strategy of radically improving value for money: quality assurance, evidence-based practice and clinical audit. Each of these will be discussed here.

Quality assurance

Quality assurance is a process designed to achieve quality services, which means striving for excellence and good practice. The aims of good practice in health have been stated as: 'to be effective, to be safe, to be efficient and to satisfy patients' (Pollock and Evans 1989, p. 21).

Quality is defined by Ellis (1988, p. 7) as 'that which gives complete customer satisfaction'. He also comments that what he terms the 'caring professions' differ from manufacturing industry from whence quality assurance arose. Instead of producing a product that is consistent, quality services are those that suit the individual requirements of patients and clients. Assurance, on the other hand, means making sure that quality is maintained (Ellis 1988, p. 8). This involves a process that is designed to set standards of quality, find out if they are being achieved and take action to improve or maintain standards as necessary.

When adopting a quality model, most purchasers of health care use one proposed by Maxwell (1984) which incorporates six dimensions:

- accessibility
- relevance to need
- equity
- social acceptability
- efficiency
- effectiveness

An alternative model from Canada, where quality management had been part of their health care scene for many years, is described by Ovretveit

(1992) who suggests that quality in health must include three dimensions:

- client quality – what clients and carers want from the service;
- professional quality – whether the service meets needs as defined by professional providers and reformers, and whether it correctly carries out techniques and procedures that are believed to be necessary to meet client needs;
- management quality – the most efficient and productive use of resources within limits and directives set by higher authorities or purchasers.

Evidence-based practice

Measuring precisely the impact that different interventions, or treatments, have on an individual's or population's health status is problematic. Is it possible to design measures that will tell us accurately the effects that our interventions are having? In reality, many of the practices used in health have never been evaluated for effectiveness.

Evidence-based practice has been defined as 'the process of systematically funding, appraising, and using contemporaneous research findings as the basis for clinical decisions' (Rosenberg and Donald 1995). A four-stage model is suggested:

- formulate a clear clinical question from a patient's problem;
- search the literature for relevant clinical articles (evidence);
- evaluate (critically appraise) the evidence for its validity and usefulness;
- implement useful findings in clinical practice.

This model helps to increase the speed of knowledge transfer from research into practice and to ensure that decisions are made on the basis of up-to-date and appropriate research evidence, rather than custom and practice experience (Long 1997).

In pursuit of the evidence-based approach, one must remember that the findings of research must be tailored to suit local circumstances before they can be incorporated into everyday practice. In addition to this, Long (1997) states 'that movement is needed towards outcomes-orientated practice, which is needs-led and patient-centred.'

Clinical audit

Audit is defined in the Government Paper 'Working for Patients' as: 'the systematic, critical analysis of the quality of medical care, including the procedures used for diagnosis and treatment, the use of resources, and the resulting outcome and quality of life for the patient' (HMSO 1990, p. 3). Audit can therefore be an important part of the quality-assurance process, aimed at finding out what is being achieved, including the outcomes. Clinical audit can be used to investigate and improve many aspects of clinical care, such as access, equity, appropriateness, acceptability, effectiveness and efficiency. Many of these quality areas need process measures, with the last two needing measures of outcome.

For the purposes of clinical audit, a service may be viewed as having three aspects: structure, process and outcome (Ellis 1988; Pollock and Evans 1989; Scottish Home and Health Department 1988). These can be defined as:

- structure – the factors affecting the material, social or intellectual environment of care;
- process – the activities required to be undertaken to provide appropriate care;
- outcome – the objectives for the results of care;

The last definition links outcomes directly to objectives but outcomes may be different from the initial objectives of therapy, and can be defined as the result of process: 'An outcome is the result of an activity' (Training Agency 1988, p. 6).

All healthcare services need to be able to measure the results of what they do as well as measure the cost of the results. However, the outcomes of occupational therapy, and other services that approach individual clients in a holistic manner, are difficult to capture. Many of the definitions used for outcomes of health care imply that they may include subjective data that cannot be measured by observation. This is especially true in areas where the goal of healthcare is not merely curative but includes holistic care. Today, the challenge is to develop measures that can be used to assess the behaviour, attitudes and feelings of people, their functional performance and changes in their interaction with other people.

Health outcomes for occupational therapists

The outcomes of occupational therapy are both difficult to determine and difficult to measure (Blom-Cooper 1989). If outcomes are defined only as items of observable behaviour, some effects of intervention may be missed because they are subjective feelings and thoughts. A second problem is that it may be difficult to be specific about desired outcomes at the start of treatment. It is often hard to find out what client's objectives are, especially if he or she has communication difficulties or is withdrawn, confused or psychotic. Initial goals for therapy may be tentative and vague, such as the therapist aiming to establish some kind of rapport with the client. The evaluation and measurement of goal attainment can be difficult if goals are vague or global. A third problem is that occupational therapists are often concerned with the direction of change rather than with defined and measurable outcomes. For example, the therapist may look for improvement in a specific functional skill without necessarily seeking to obtain full function. It is hard to measure outcomes when goals have been couched in vague terms such as 'partial improvement'.

In the past, it has been thought that occupational therapists cannot evaluate their practice effectively because we do not have the skills in quantitative research. However, it may be that these are not the right tools because our outcomes cannot easily be quantified. Occupational therapists use a variety of frames of reference and often mix theories and approaches. The profession does not have a single, focused theoretical perspective on which to draw, with its own convention of research methods (as in medicine). If occupational therapy is not a science it must be an art, which will not be measurable by scientific methods.

In defining the term 'outcome', one can differentiate between a predetermined outcome and an outcome meaning the actual results of therapy. The usefulness of setting specific therapy goals is well recognised, as is measuring predetermined outcomes to give what appear to be concrete and tangible criteria to use as evidence of effectiveness. However, there is concern that predetermined outcomes reveal only part of the story. Cook (1991, p. 12) discusses her own concerns about an anxiety management course. The objective of the course was for participants to learn skills and knowledge that would enable them to reduce their high levels of anxiety and the frequency of panic attacks. On completion of the course, one member said that a significant outcome for her had been that she had met and made a new friend. She described this developing relationship as having improved her quality of life, yet it had not been a predetermined outcome of therapy.

The problems with predetermined outcomes are that they do not provide a valid test of effectiveness because they do not include other outcomes that were not originally predicted, and they are not reliable because it is difficult to predict accurately the extent and level to which a client is able to respond to any particular therapeutic process.

How occupational therapists are tackling outcome measurement

The first step towards effective outcome measurement is to establish a baseline from which to measure change. It is necessary to be clear about the level at which the client is starting, as well as the level he or she is aiming for. In order to clarify and define the level of outcome that is expected, the therapist needs to include information about:

- the patient's activities and behaviour, including the performance of skills, range of abilities, level of function and social behaviour;
- the patient's feelings and attitudes;
- the degree of knowledge and understanding the patient has;

- the amount and type of assistance needed to perform tasks, including equipment, physical assistance and physical or verbal prompting;
- the length of time taken to complete tasks and the frequency of performance;
- features of the environment, including adaptations.

Once the baseline has been established, desired outcomes can be determined. These may be expressed as behavioural objectives. Behavioural objectives are much harder to set than goals couched in terms of direction of change or subjective experience, but they are much easier to measure. For example, it is easier to assess objectively a change in observable behaviour than a subjective change such as 'feeling more confident'. A behaviour is the performance of an observable function at a specific level in a specified situation. The behaviour may be observed before treatment is implemented and after intervention and can be used as an indicator of the desired change in function.

For an outcome to be measurable, specifications are needed such as target behaviour, level of performance, equipment needed and environment. Non-observable constructs such as self concept, which seem unmeasurable, can be operationalised to provide indicators of change which can be measured (Anton 1978). Operationalisation consists of the therapist and client selecting items of observable behaviour that they would expect to change in relation to internal subjective changes.

Ottenbacher and Cusick (1988) argue that the vagueness of occupational therapy goals and the related predetermined outcomes can be corrected using a system called 'goal attainment scaling' to evaluate the outcome of programmes with individual clients. Goals are transformed into specific items of behaviour that can be measured, in a way similar to the operationalisation of constructs. However, setting the expected level of performance for any goal 'is based on the assumption that experienced clinical practitioners will be able to predict treatment outcomes with information from the client, family members, and other health care providers' (Ottenbacher and Cusick 1988, p. 521). Lack of reliability concerning prediction can be a limitation, that may need 'extensive training' to overcome (Ottenbacher and Cusick 1988, p. 520). Despite its limitations, goal attainment scaling does seem to represent an improvement over subjective and anecdotal evaluation.

An additional benefit of translating subjective goals into observable behaviours is that the operationalised indicator could become a useful symbolic action for the client, as illustrated in this case study.

Case example 1

A client became overwhelmed with unresolved grief after the death of her first baby and two of her grandparents. The goals that she negotiated with the therapist were:

- to express her feelings and develop strategies that would provide her with safe opportunities to express her feelings;
- to revisit her baby's grave;
- to externalise her grief by planting a tree in memory of her baby.

The symbolic ritual of tree planting is an item of behaviour that was used as a marker that the woman had reached some acceptance of her grief through having the opportunity to express it in counselling sessions.

The tool used to measure outcomes will be selected to suit the type of change being measured. For physiological changes, such as those sought in problems of weight, heart rate or incontinence, it may be necessary to take measurements with biomedical instruments. The client, carer, therapist or other staff could do this. Changes in observable behaviour, such as problems of function or communication, or changes in the environment or equipment, may be observed and reported by client, carer, therapist and other staff. Subjective changes, such as changes in level of confidence, acceptance of disability or degree of pain, must be reported by the client unless they are operationalised into observable items of behaviour that reflect the changes.

This case example, of a client who had become socially isolated, shows how subjective changes were operationalised into items of behaviour that could be measured objectively.

Case example 2

A client was attending a mental health unit on an outpatient basis and participating in an anxiety management programme. This was not the first time she has been through the programme.

The client was asked what she would do differently if she felt different. She replied, 'Well, if I felt more confident I think I would say something to my new neighbour. I keep on seeing her but I don't actually say hello.'

This behavioural outcome (talking to her new neighbour) was chosen by the client to indicate attainment of the subjective outcome she wanted to achieve (feeling less anxious). An agreed indicator was attached to the goal to show how the change was to be measured. Thus the desired outcome became:

- Goal: to improve confidence in talking with people.
- Indicator: to initiate a conversation with my neighbour.

Individualised outcome measurement

The profession as a whole has adopted two main methods of capturing the outcomes of occupational therapy interventions. These are standardised and individualised outcome measurements. Examples of standardised measures are the SF36 (Garratt et al. 1993), which is a health profile, and the Bartel Index (Wade 1992). These measures have been tested for reliability and validity over large populations and the scores are published, allowing therapists to compare results with each other. They also allow a client's scores to be compared to a normal range and to other clients with similar conditions. Measures such as the SF-36 merely collect information from patients but do not take into account additional factors, such as their own desired goals of treatment.

For many professionals working within a multi-professional team, with clients who often have multiple pathologies, treatments and outcomes do not follow standardised formats. Individualised programmes of care, designed to meet each individual's needs, will result in variations in the desired outcomes related closely to that client's social, psychological and emotional needs. This means that success cannot be standardised for any one group of clients but the focus of intervention is on attaining goals or resolving problems that are particularly important to a particular person. Individualised measures are more sensitive to small changes that may be important to the client. However, as Cook (1991) states, outcome measures do need to reflect any variation between desired and expected outcomes for individuals.

Examples of individualised outcome measurement tools include:

- treatment evaluation by Le Roux's Method (TELER) (Le Roux 1993);
- goal attainment scaling (Ottenbacher and Cusick 1990);
- Canadian Occupational Performance Measure (COPM) (Law et al. 1991).

All these measures are scaled. They can be used for all client groups and allow for very specific outcomes to be measured.

Individualised outcome measures capture what it is that the client wants out of therapy and what therapists achieve in day-to-day practice. They have good face and content validity and are responsive to change. However, as each client's goals are different, it is difficult to ensure that achievement is being measured the same way across many clients. In order to work towards more reliable and comparable measurement, it is helpful for groups of staff to discuss individual cases and to question each other about how they are setting expected outcomes and managing actual outcomes.

There are three stages in applying individualised outcome measures:

- Individual problems or goals are identified and negotiated with the client. These indicate the expected outcomes of therapy.
- A programme of therapy is planned and implemented.
- Following an agreed time limit of therapy or number of sessions, actual achieved outcomes are compared to the expected outcome to measure whether therapy has been effective.

The usefulness of setting specific therapy goals and measuring the extent to which they have been reached is well recognised within the therapy professions. Predetermined outcomes give concrete and tangible criteria to use as evidence of the effectiveness of a particular intervention. When the approach to treatment planning is client centred, goals or problems are negotiated with both client and carer. This ensures that the client is an active participant in the therapy process and is more able to understand and measure the changes that take place. It also helps to ensure that the purpose of therapy is driven by the client rather than by the therapist or multi-professional team.

It may be that the team or therapist do not agree to work towards all of the clients' goals because of reasons of safety, professional knowledge or ethics. This should be stated explicitly in the client's documentation and may also be used in a therapy contract. It may become apparent that the carer has goals that are conflicting or separate from those of the client, and these also need negotiating. Sometimes, in a multi-professional team, it is possible to bring in a co-worker to work with the carer, for example a social worker or advocate.

The following case example illustrates a set of goals for a parent and child that includes changes in feelings, attitudes and performance.

Case example 3

Jim is a child with cerebral palsy, attending a Child Development Centre on an outpatient basis. Goals have been set for a period of treatment lasting for three months and they will be reviewed at the end of this time. They are:

- for Jim to hold a spoon on his own;
- for Jim's mother to feel less anxious at meal times;
- for Jim's mother to allow him to eat with the family at the table;
- for Jim's mother to allow him a 15-minute trial period feeding himself at meal times.

The first goal concerns the child's function. The second goal is subjective for Jim's mother. The other two goals describe changes in the mother's behaviour that will result from changes in her feelings and attitudes.

When working with clients who have communication, perceptive or cognitive difficulties, or who are unable to make decisions, the therapist or team may set the initial goals or define the initial problems. These may focus on enabling the client to express their needs and wants and to make decisions. This is an important stage in the process of encouraging autonomy, self-worth and self-advocacy.

In fields such as paediatrics and mental health, focusing on problems is seen as too negative, whereas 'goal' is a word better suited both to client and carer. Many people working in acute, physical fields and with the elderly find that problems fit the common language of their clients; for example, it is a common opening line to ask 'what problems are you experiencing at home?'

There is some concern that the process of negotiating goals and problems may make some clients feel under pressure or set them up to fail. This may be the case when a time limit is put on the therapy. Clients who have been through therapy a number times may not have encountered a time limit before. However, the process of negotiating goals and problems is also therapeutic. It gives clients encouragement, provided that achievable goals are set. Often, in areas of mental health, clients who live in chaotic environments see this process as a step to helping them to achieve some sort of order. Time may be measured in terms of days, weeks, months or number of sessions required for the outcome to be attained. Review dates or times are also required for maintenance goals.

The following case example illustrates how a client and therapist worked together to set short-term goals as part of the therapeutic process.

Case example 4

The client was suffering from a high level of anxiety and the therapist spent several sessions building up his trust and confidence. This resulted in two goals that were decided together:

- the client would produce a list of goals;
- the client would update his relaxation skills and carry out relaxation on his own.

He achieved both of these and produced the following hierarchy of goals (from the least threatening to the most threatening):

- going fishing
- going to a football match
- meeting friends
- phoning friends to arrange to go out
- playing football in the local team
- visiting a friend's house
- attending a job interview
- going to the pub with friends
- going on a date with a girl.

Having negotiated the goals of therapy, therapists and clients require a way of evaluating the results (outcomes) of the therapy programme.

The simplest method of measuring achievements is a binary method (Cook and Spreadbury 1995) – that is, the expected outcome has been achieved or not. This is then scored as 'yes' (+1) or 'no' (0).

In order to trust the results of a binary individualised outcome measure, the therapist has to feel confident that the measure is sensitive, valid and reliable. These factors rely on the skill with which the expected outcomes are defined, prior to an episode of therapy. Each expected outcome, whether it is resolving a problem or attaining a goal, needs to be defined as a short-term, specific, time-limited, observable, expected outcome that is achievable through the planned programme of therapy.

If the aim of therapy is to produce internal (affective and cognitive) changes as well as external (behavioural) changes in clients, and therapists cannot force these changes, then clients not only have to be willing to move in certain directions but also have to take an active part in the process of change. Therapy may, therefore, be more akin to personal learning than medical treatment. The occupational therapist offers the client opportunities to learn about herself or himself and the need for change. Further opportunities are then offered to learn the necessary skills for making that change and, often, to learn about community resources that will help to facilitate change.

Defining therapy as learning rather than treatment influences the discussion of therapy outcomes. If the client is an active participant in the process, the outcomes of therapy will be due to the input of both the therapist and the client, and not just that of the therapist. The perceptions of the client about the goals of therapy – what happens during that process and the results – are therefore very important in any efforts to understand the outcomes of occupational therapy.

As well as capturing the specific outcomes of occupational therapy there is a need for measures that could also be used with a multidisciplinary team. Initially, there was considerable speculation about whether individualised measures that were integrated with routine patient documentation could form part of a multidisciplinary system of record keeping. However, using individualised outcome measures, occupational therapists have found that the clarity of the expected outcomes helps them to define the boundaries of their role for each client's programme of therapy. This includes the limitations of roles within a multidisciplinary team and the boundaries between different agencies acting to support a client in the community.

The measurement of individualised outcomes has been shown to fit extremely well with the process of rehabilitation and to enhance clinical reasoning. The main difficulties have occurred where therapists are not used to thinking in terms of process being distinct from outcomes. A further difficulty occurs where therapists are not used to articulating the expected outcome of a programme of therapy in concise and specific wording. The development of these skills is shown to be beneficial for the professional development of staff, but it takes considerable time and effort to adopt new habits of thinking and record keeping.

Having clearly defined the expected outcomes for a client, it is then possible to compare these with the actual outcomes that result from therapy. As well as being very useful information for the planning and evaluation of individual therapy programmes, the outcome data can be audited over several clients in a service. Individualised measures of outcomes are useful for audit/service review purposes because they are suitable for client centred, holistic therapy and recognise the autonomy of the individual client. However, to use this measure, sufficient training needs to be provided, and time allocated for staff to learn and adopt it as routine.

Summary

As pressure on health services has increased, so the need to measure performance has become greater. This, coupled with an increase in the evaluation by different professional groups of the effectiveness of their interventions, has resulted in a climate of measurement and evaluation in the 1990s. The challenge for therapists has been great as they have sought appropriate tools to evaluate their work, developing, testing and, in many cases, discarding new ones.

The outcomes of occupational therapy may be:

- subjective changes as well as observable behaviour;
- goal free or non-specific as well as fulfilling predetermined specific goals;
- peculiar to individual clients rather than shared by many;
- indicative of individual priorities.

This approach to measuring individualised outcomes has been successful in defining the outcomes of a wide range of activities and treatments offered by occupational therapists. These include changes in daily living skills, mobility, use of equipment, social behaviour, knowledge, feelings and attitudes. The measurement of attitudes and feelings is most important for the holistic care that characterises the work of many people in rehabilitation. It is achieved through two mechanisms: firstly, individualising the expected outcomes of therapy and, secondly, by operationalising subjective changes into observable items of behaviour.

Individualised outcomes have proved to be one of the most popular and successful methods for measuring and improving patient care. The reason for this may be that health outcomes, especially where the intervention is not limited to a curative approach, have proved difficult to evaluate using quantitative methodologies. This applies particularly to the profession of occupational therapy, which takes a client-centred approach and is concerned with individual aspirations and goals.

Acknowledgement

The author would like to thank Sarah Cook without whose advice and help this chapter would never have been started.

References

Anton J (1978) Studying Individual Change. In Goldman L (ed.) Research Methods for Counsellors. New York: Wiley.

Blom-Cooper L (1989) Occupational Therapy, an Emerging Profession in Health Care. London: Duckworth.

Burck HD (1978) Evaluation Programs: Models and Strategies. In Goldman L (ed.) Research Methods for Counsellors. New York: Wiley.

Cook SA (1991) A Study of the Outcomes of Occupational Therapy In Mental Health Services. Unpublished M.Ed dissertation. Sheffield: Hallam University.

Cook S, Spreadbury P (1995) Measuring the Outcomes of Individualised Care: the Binary Individualised Outcome Measure. Nottingham: Nottingham City Hospital NHS Trust.

Ellis R (1988) Quality Assurance and Care. In Professional Competence and Quality Assurance in the Caring Professions. London: Croom Helm.

Garratt AM, Ruta DA, Abdulla MI, Buckingham JK, Russell IT (1993) The SF 36 health survey questionnaire: an outcome measure suitable for routine use within the NHS? British Medical Journal 2(9): 349–51.

Goble R (1989) Research in occupational therapy: luxury or necessity? British Journal of Occupational Therapy 52(9): 349–51.

Griffiths R (1983) NHS Management Inquiry. London: HMSO.

Gudex C (1986) QALYs and their Use in the Health Service. Discussion paper No. 20. York: Centre for Health Economics, York University.

HMSO (1990) Medical Audit, Working Paper 6. Working for Patients, Cm 555. London: HMSO.

Koch J (1991) Quality Management in Healthcare. London: Longman.

Le Roux A (1993) TELER the concept. Journal of Physiotherapy 79(11): 755–85.

Long AF (1997) Evidence Based Practice at a Managerial and Clinical Practice Level Background paper: Session 1, Internal Symposium ECHHO, Linkoping, Sweden, 12–13 June.

Law M, Baptiste S, Caswell A, McColl MA, Polatajiko H, Pollock N (1994) Canadian Occupational Performance Measure 2nd ed. Toronto: CAOT Publications

Maxwell RJ (1984) Quality assessment in health. British Medical Journal 288 (May) 1470–7.

Ottenbacher K, Cusack A (1988) The significance of clinical change and clinical change of significance: issues and methods. American Journal of Occupational Therapy 44(6): 519–25.

Ovretveit J (1992) Health Service Quality: and introduction to quality methods for health services. Oxford: Blackwell Scientific Publications.

Pollock A, Evans M (1989) Surgical Audit. London: Butterworths.

Rosenberg W, Donald A (1995) Evidence-based medicine: an approach to clinical problem solving. British Medical Journal 310: 1122–6.

Scottish Home and Health Department (1988) Quality Assurance in Nursing. Edinburgh: HMSO.

Strong P, Robinson J (1988) New Model Management: Griffiths and the NHS. Warwick: Nursing Policy Studies Centre, University of Warwick.

Training Agency (1988) Development of Assessable Standards for National Certification. Sheffield: Training Agency.

Wade DT (1992) Measurement in Neurological Rehabilitation. Oxford: Oxford University Press.

Chapter 8
Communicating the nature and purpose of occupational therapy

JENNIFER CREEK

Introduction

Occupational therapists have difficulty putting what they do into words. This is not a new problem or one that is confined to the UK; it has been mentioned in the occupational therapy literature around the world for many years and is still being widely discussed. Schön (1983, p. 49) suggested that all practice professions have difficulty in saying what they do because so much of their knowledge is tacit, 'a kind of knowing in practice'. However, occupational therapists seem to be particularly concerned about who and what they are. They appear to suffer from a weak sense of professional identity and chronic uncertainty about their role and function, which is, in some way, connected to their difficulties with language.

The first section of this chapter reviews what has been written in the occupational therapy literature about the problematic relationship the profession has with language. Three manifestations of the problem are identified: difficulty defining occupational therapy, failure to agree on the meanings of key professional concepts and difficulty explaining the role and function of occupational therapists. The second section explores the problem in greater depth, looking at the precise nature of the difficulties occupational therapists have with language. The final section considers possible reasons for these difficulties. Two theories are used to give a perspective from which the problem can be understood. These are linguistic theory and post-modern feminist theory. Linguistic theory is used to illuminate why occupational therapists, who use high-level communication skills in their work, cannot communicate effectively the nature and purpose of that work. Postmodern feminist theory is used to explore the relationships between the mainly female composition of the profession, the feminine nature of the job, the masculine systems and structures within which occupational therapists work and the gendered nature of language.

Occupational therapists' problem with language

The difficulty occupational therapists have in articulating their purpose and function can be seen to manifest itself in three ways in the literature of the profession:

* there is no clear and generally accepted definition of occupational therapy;
* there is disagreement about how key professional concepts should be defined;
* occupational therapists are not able to define with certainty their role and function in the many fields in which they practise.

Defining occupational therapy

For many years occupational therapists have lamented the lack of a clear definition of occupational therapy that will tell the world, and themselves, what they are and what they do. They complain of 'widespread and persistent misconcepts about the practice and purpose of occupational therapy' (Dunkin and Goble 1982, p. 46), which they ascribe to not being able to tell people what they are doing. It seems that the nature and function of occupational therapy are not self-evident.

Mocellin (1988, p. 4) commented that 'in any discussion on the lack of public awareness about occupational therapy and the poor identity and self-esteem that many occupational therapists seem to have about themselves, little emphasis is usually placed on the definition of occupational therapy as a potential remedy for some of these problems.' Mocellin is mistaken. Occupational therapists worldwide have persistently sought a clear definition of the profession and continue to do so.

In the UK, Green (1977, p. 300) stated that 'A definition of occupational therapy is badly needed and it is badly needed for three reasons. These are: 1. that occupational therapists should practise effectively; 2. that concepts can be taught to students, and a rationale explained to outsiders; 3. that practice may be evaluated and developed.' Hall (1989, p. 244) noted that 'problems [within occupational therapy] are thought to stem from having an unclear professional identity and no clearly defined body of knowledge or theory of occupational therapy.' Hollis (1993) suggested that unless occupational therapists can define themselves they remain vulnerable to being defined by the organisations that employ them.

In the USA, Shannon (1977, p. 230) commented that 'Occupational therapy cannot be defined descriptively (what it is), nor is there agreement on a normative definition (what it ought to be).' Engelhardt (1977) gave three reasons for seeking a definition of the profession: to become clearer about the values that structure and guide practice; to answer critics of the medicalisation of human life; and to justify having an independent profession of occupational therapy. Clark (1979, p. 506) warned that 'other professions are usurping therapists' jobs because occupational therapy has been unable to clearly define its role, function and theoretical and research bases.' Yerxa et al. (1989, p. 2) complained that 'Occupational therapists in clinical practice are told, often by business managers, to explain and justify what they do'.

In Australia, Goode (1956, cited by Bell 1991, p. 22) wrote of the need to 'define what we are doing, clarify our thinking.' Mocellin (1984) claimed that the greatest challenge to occupational therapists is to be able 'to communicate what they do and how their services will benefit people.' Bell (1991, p. 128) suggested that 'from its beginnings . . . occupational therapy has had difficulty projecting an image and defining what the profession does' and felt that, in 1991, 'we are still being challenged to define our professional role succinctly and clearly to others' (p. 130).

In Israel, Sachs and Jarus (1992) spoke of 'difficulties in defining the profession as a whole, its roles and especially its boundaries.'

Not being able to say clearly what occupational therapy is means that it cannot be explained to other people. Significant others include: those who receive occupational therapy intervention; those who may choose to buy, or in other ways support, occupational therapy services; referring agents; the other professionals we work with; potential students; health policy makers, and the general public.

A small study carried out within a psychiatric teaching hospital, in 1992, found that the reasons doctors gave for referring people to occupational therapy were very vague and concluded that 'The doctors were unclear about occupational therapy as a tool and . . . found it difficult to give clear cut reasons for referral' (Sheik and Boultan 1992, p. 407). Engelhardt (1977, p. 670) lamented that occupational therapists cannot attract public attention and funds in the same way that those seeking funding for the cure of cancer can, because 'Most persons are more fearful of cancer than desirous of good occupational therapy.' He went on to argue that people need to be convinced that enterprises which try to enrich the breadth of human life, such as occupational therapy, are more important than those that increase its length. Part of the problem is that the goal of enriching life is a complex one, and difficult to grasp, whereas the goal of prolonging life is simple to communicate and easy to understand.

Defining key professional concepts

Hagedorn (1995, p. 13) claimed that 'Words are important . . . Precision in language is necessary, and it is essential for a profession to have an agreed vocabulary, avoiding the use of jargon.' However, this precision has not yet been achieved in occupational therapy.

Nelson (1988) spoke of the ambiguity of the key words used by occupational therapists, such as occupation, activity, play and work. He suggested that such ambiguity can inhibit the development of the profession and emphasised the need to define terms accurately in order to ensure that everyone knows exactly what is being discussed. Breines (1995), on the other hand, argued that the term 'occupation' is especially useful because it is both ambiguous and comprehensive. 'The diverse ways in which occupation can be defined suggests that this term is extraordinarily comprehensive. Moreover, precisely because of this comprehensiveness, occupation has evaded unique definition' (p. 459). Breines' contention was that the breadth, diversity and complexity of occupational therapy practice can only be captured by a term that holds various meanings and encapsulates all aspects of the profession. This still leaves the problem of knowing which meaning is intended in any particular situation.

Katz and Sachs (1991) claimed that not only do occupational therapists define key professional concepts in a variety of ways but they also attribute different levels of importance to them. The definitions and their levels of importance represent the ideology of occupational therapy; therefore, clarification of meanings can contribute to an understanding of occupational therapy, both among occupational therapists from different cultures and between professionals and non-professionals. Not being able to define key professional concepts can lead to intra- and interdisciplinary confusion.

When words are used that have not been given a meaning specific to occupational therapy, they are open to misinterpretation. This applies to the everyday words used by occupational therapists, such as 'activity', as well as to the technical terms borrowed from other disciplines, such as 'behaviour'. The general public does not understand how activity can be used as a treatment medium. Other professions are likely to interpret what occupational therapists say about their work in the light of their own theories and definitions. Occupational therapists themselves remain unclear about who they are, what they do, where their professional domain of concern lies and how occupational therapy theory and practice are different from those of other professions.

The role and function of occupational therapists

Occupational therapists appear to be very concerned about defining their clinical role. Barris (1984) wrote that, from the 1960s onwards, role diffusion and confusion was evident in the profession as demonstrated by the 'proliferation of journal articles . . . calling for reorganization of the field's existing knowledge; from surveys of occupational therapy practices revealing inconsistencies and difficulties in rationalizing treatment approaches; and from continuing conflicts and debates over potential "new" models of practice' (p. 5). Barris linked role confusion with a tendency to develop knowledge and expertise in specialist areas without concurrently strengthening the generic knowledge base of the profession.

A study carried out in Israel (Sachs and Jarus 1992) found that occupational therapists did not feel recognised and appreciated by their professional colleagues. They had to explain repeatedly to physicians and other professionals how occupational therapy can help patients. This study also suggested that occupational therapists working in the fields of psychiatry and the care of the elderly have more difficulty defining the boundaries of their role than occupational therapists in other fields. This was ascribed to the strong holistic basis of practice in these areas.

Green (1991, p. 53) wrote that 'It appears that occupational therapy is suffering from a chronic case of role anxiety which, if neglected, could have serious consequences. It is manifest on an international as well as a national scale and it has been with us for some time.'

In the *British Journal of Occupational Therapy*, in the 10 years from 1984 to 1993, 45 articles were published in which the major focus was the role of the occupational therapist in a particular setting. The occupational therapist's role was examined in two ways: the role with specific disabilities, for example, cardiac rehabilitation, bone marrow transplants and AIDS; and the role in an area of practice or treatment setting, such as a psychotherapy unit, community mental health or the primary health care team.

Failure to define clearly the role and function of occupational therapy within particular practice settings means that occupational therapists are under constant threat from other professions trying to take over aspects of their work. They are often seen as 'jacks of all trades and masters of none' because of the diversity of their work (Bell 1991, p. 128) and it is easy to think that most of the functions of the occupational therapist could be carried out by other professionals. Colleagues see the commonplace, everyday activities which occupational therapists use as treatment methods and may confuse them with the goals of intervention. Getting the client to make a cup of tea or weave a basket is not the goal but the means towards more complex goals. The casual observer might think that anyone could run a current affairs discussion group or take a cookery session but the same observer might lack awareness of the factors that make these activities therapeutic.

Boundary disputes are an everyday part of the occupational therapist's working life and, without a language of occupational therapy, it is difficult to define boundaries and defend territory.

Failing to communicate

The previous section identified how occupational therapists view their own attempts to communicate the nature and purpose of what they do. This section explores in more depth the precise nature of occupational therapists' problems in finding a universally accepted definition of occupational therapy, agreeing on the meaning of key professional concepts and explaining occupational therapy to others.

Why occupational therapy is difficult to define

The *Concise Oxford Dictionary* defined definition as 'Stating precise nature of thing or meaning of word; form of words in which this is done; making or being distinct.' To define a word is to state its meaning.

The difficulty that occupational therapists have in finding a satisfactory definition of occupational therapy has been expressed by several writers, for example:

> The role, identity and theory of occupational therapy are not easy to define specifically. There may be confusion and disagreement over what occupational therapy is and does. (Busuttil 1992, p. 461)

> To formulate any definition is indeed an exercise in semantics . . . To formulate a definition of Occupational Therapy for Occupational Therapists is an even more overwhelming task especially as one is not always sure that we all see Occupational Therapy through the same telescope. (Du Toit 1979, p. 429)

> Official definitions of occupational therapy appear to either give vague generic statements or define occupational therapy specifically in one setting. This leaves individuals to decide whether to use one or other approach or a combination of the two. (Lycett 1991, p. 411)

Part of the problem lies in expressing the nature of occupational therapy succinctly. Reed and Sanderson (1980) claimed that, in order to be useful in today's world, a definition of a profession must include a brief account of the unique features of the profession; the major professional goals; the population served; a summary of the services offered; the process of intervention; and the techniques, media or method used. In addition, all of these must be expressed concisely. Blom-Cooper (1989, p. 14) found existing definitions of occupational therapy in the UK 'too broad and unfocused to be useful'.

Another problem in defining occupational therapy seems to be the breadth of practice, which makes it almost impossible for occupational therapists in different fields to agree on what they have in common that could be used to define the uniqueness of the profession. MacDonald (1960, quoted by Woods 1990a, p. 471) described occupational therapy as 'a treatment service which has so many facets and so few boundaries.' Sachs and Jarus (1992) stated that 'The broad professional definition and professional diversity results sometimes in a large number of responsibilities for the practitioners and in difficulties in defining the profession as a whole.' MacDonald (1990, p. 341) suggested that a variety of definitions is needed for different applications, and that there is skill in being able to expand and interpret definitions 'to enlighten the audience being addressed'.

A third problem is that occupational therapy is changing all the time so that even if a definition could be agreed for current use it would no longer be adequate in a few years time. Du Toit (1979, p. 429) suggested that 'With the continuous growth of the profession, original definitions become outdated and we need to periodically confirm that we still speak the same Occupational Therapy language.' Wheeler (1972, quoted by Woods 1990b, p. 471) warned against attempting to 'freeze the occupational therapy image solid once and for all'. Woods (1990a, p. 248) expressed dissatisfaction with current definitions of occupational therapy, on the grounds that they tended to be 'a little too medically orientated, and unable to embrace the range of current professional practice.'

The name 'occupational therapy' itself is felt by many therapists to be misleading in the impression of the profession it gives to others. Occupational therapy was adopted as a title by the profession in the USA, in 1915, when occupational therapists had a very distinct purpose in providing structured programmes of useful activity for people confined to institutions for long periods of time. At that time, it may be assumed, the name conveyed the meaning of the concept adequately. In the 80 years since the name came into use, occupational therapy has expanded into many different countries and many different areas of practice. The purpose and practice of occupational therapy are not only different from what they were in 1915 but also vary from country to country, from field of practice to field of practice, from one therapist to another and from one client to another.

There is evidence that practitioners today feel that the term 'occupational therapy' is no longer an adequate signifier – that is, it does not convey the meaning of the profession. Many occupational therapists have written, in articles or letters to their professional journals, that we should change our name. Horner (1983, p. 237) wrote that she 'would welcome a more appropriate title'. Clark et al. (1991, p. 301) complained that:

We are tired of trying to describe what occupational therapists do, of seeing one article after another extolling the virtues of occupation (whatever it is), and of hearing lectures that promise once and for all to clarify the meaning of the term occupation. Some of us, in fact, think that if we could just delete the word occupational from the name of the profession, we would be far better off.

The name 'occupational therapy' is perceived to be linked with an outdated image of the profession that was appropriate at one time but is no longer so. Our meaning seems to have been fixed at the time when we worked in institutions, so that many people think of occupational therapists as craft ladies. The press is still reinforcing this image. For example, a comment in an article in the *Guardian* newspaper (Moncur 1994) implied that occupational therapy is something of a joke, not a healthcare profession to be taken seriously:

> I am launching a new pressure group, to be known for short as SFTRFCOADCWRABSBYDAIOT. That's the Society For The Removal From Churches Of Any Duff Craftwork Which Resembles A Bedspread Stitched By Your Dotty Aunt In Occupational Therapy.

The report of an independent commission of inquiry into occupational therapy in the UK, published in 1989, commented adversely on the profession's title:

> Some of the evidence we obtained during the course of our inquiry confirmed the persistence of outdated stereotypes of what the profession's work entailed in sharp distinction to the activities in which its members were actually engaged. Such stereotypes are undoubtedly a handicap to a proper regard for the status of the profession and an appreciation of the value of the work actually performed by occupational therapists. So much so indeed that we felt that the very title 'occupational therapy' could partially account for its remaining, despite a substantial growth in its numbers and far-reaching tributes to the value of their contribution, a 'submerged' profession. (Blom-Cooper 1989, p. 17)

Occupational therapists have not succeeded in changing the meaning of their title so that it signifies the present-day profession, rather than that of the turn of the century. Other professions have done this. The profession of medicine, for example, is very different from what it was 100 years ago and yet people now understand the up-to-date meaning of the term doctor as well as people in the last century understood the meaning that it held then. Doctors have succeeded in changing the meaning of medicine, but occupational therapists have not succeeded in changing the meaning of occupational therapy.

Occupational therapy terminology

The profession of occupational therapy began as a practice-based profession directed by physicians. The early occupational therapists did not have their own theories to tell them how and when to intervene, or to explain why what they did worked or did not work. They depended on the medical profession to provide a theoretical underpinning to what they did, and so they did not need their own concepts or words to name those concepts. The methods of intervention that occupational therapists used were the activities of everyday life and did not require special names to refer to them. A physiotherapist might call her treatment technique 'gait re-education', but the occupational therapist could say that she got the client to 'make a cup of tea'. Occupational therapists used both the activities and the language of everyday life.

As the profession of occupational therapy developed, practitioners began to use theories for themselves, but these were theories borrowed and adapted from other disciplines, such as the classification of diseases from medicine and theories of motivation from psychology. Along with theories, occupational therapy adopted the concepts underpinning those theories and the terminology used to communicate them. In the past three decades, occupational therapists have made progress in formulating their own views of people, dysfunction and remediation, but a large part of their theory base still comes from other disciplines.

The development of the profession has left occupational therapists with two problems. The first is that much of our language has been adopted from other disciplines and has meanings that those disciplines have ascribed to it. For example, we have taken the term depression from psychiatry to refer to a cluster of signs and symptoms that include low mood, psychomotor retardation, loss of volition and feelings of guilt and unworthiness. This term, with its implication of a discrete condition and its medical connotations of pathology and curability, does not convey the sense that occupational therapists have of very different conditions in different individuals. Occupational therapists know that some cases of depression are closely connected with what people do in their daily lives and are therefore subject, in many cases, to amelioration through changing the way that people spend their time.

The second problem is that, whereas occupational therapists have been developing complicated theories to explain and predict the results of the use of activity as treatment, they still use the simple activities of everyday life as treatment techniques. Reilly (1962, p. 1) commented on 'the wide and gaping chasm which exists between the complexity of illness and the commonplaceness of our treatment tools'. There does not seem to be any point in trying to give a technical name to the process of making a cup of tea. However, occupational therapists do need to find their own names for the concepts that make up their professional world view in order to be able to communicate the complexity of under-standing that underlies the simplicity of what we do.

Certain concepts are widely used in occupational therapy and are generally agreed to be central to an understanding of what occupational therapy is about. Katz and Sachs (1991) identified six concepts basic to occupational therapy: function, doing, purposeful activity, occupation, work/play and leisure. They pointed out that 'The definitions of these concepts vary, however, throughout the occupational therapy literature, and usually one or more of them are used to define another concept. Moreover, each of the profession's theoretical approaches emphasises different concepts, defines them in different ways and argues their importance over the use of other concepts' (Katz and Sachs 1991, p. 137). Mosey (1985, p. 507) stated that occupational therapists lack a common vocabulary. 'Everyone has their own definition for a particular term, has no definition at all, or uses the same term to label very different concepts.'

Each occupational therapy writer defines terms differently or offers a variety of definitions and leaves the reader to choose which one she prefers. For example, the word occupation is central to the profession and yet there is no agreement on what it means. Polatajko (1992, p. 191) said that 'Occupation has neither a specific nor precise meaning – it has several meanings.' Nelson (1988, p. 633) described occupation as an ambiguous term.

A multiplicity of meanings is not the only problem that occupational therapists have with key words. Some concepts, by their nature, appear to defy definition. For example, the phrase 'purposeful activity' is sometimes used to refer to the main tool for intervention that occupational therapists use. Breines (1984, p. 543) pointed out that it is difficult to define purposeful activity 'except in terms of the individual . . . purposeful activity cannot be defined by one individual for any other individual . . . It is a personal construction, which is solely dependent on individual choice and subject to the influence of the structural and personal environment of the individual.' Occupational therapists can neither define nor prescribe purposeful activity for their clients.

A third problem that appears with occupational therapy terminology is failure to produce any adequate definition at all of particular concepts. For example, a word that is widely used when referring to the goals of occupational therapy is 'function'. Unsworth (1993, p. 287) wrote that, 'An individual's ability to function is the basis for most occupational therapy practice,' but she went on to point out that, 'in many cases, function is inappropriately defined as being what functional assessments measure.' The failure to be clear about what is meant by function can lead to functional assessments being 'dangerously inadequate'.

While many of the basic concepts of occupational therapy are borrowed and have names that are not unique to the profession, there are other concepts that are part of the theories being developed by occupational therapists. It might be expected that the names given to these concepts will be less problematic. Examples of these concepts include occupational behaviour (Reilly 1969), occupational performance (Mosey 1986), human occupation (Kielhofner and Burke 1980) and occupational science (Yerxa et al. 1990). It is interesting to note that, whereas occupational therapists deplore their profession's title and seek a name that does not include the word 'occupation', they have used this word to name so many major new concepts.

The *Concise Oxford Dictionary* defined occupation as: 'what occupies one, means of passing one's time, temporary or regular employment, business, calling, pursuit'. This is not the meaning that occupational therapists give the word. Polatajko (1992, p. 191) said that 'the meaning occupational therapists ascribe to the term "occupation" is neither the common meaning of the term nor is our meaning shared with most non-occupational therapists.' Wilcock (1993, p. 200) emphasised that 'Occupation is a central aspect of human experience, being much more, despite current usage of the word, than paid employment.' Yerxa (1993, p. 5) defined occupations as: 'units of activity which are classified and named by the culture according to the purposes they serve in enabling people to meet environmental challenges successfully.'

The other words used in these four names are equally problematic. Behaviour is a term borrowed from the discipline of psychology where it is given a precise, technical meaning: 'The total response, motor and glandular, which an organism makes to any situation with which it is faced' (Drever 1952). Occupational therapists may have their own understanding of the term, but other professionals will be more familiar with its psychological meaning. Performance is a term borrowed from role theory, used in the discipline of sociology. Nelson (1988) made a contribution to giving this term a meaning specific to occupational therapy when he elucidated the difference between the form of an occupation (a pre-existing format that guides human doing) and the performance of an occupation (the actual doing by an individual). However, there is no evidence that this clarification of meaning has gone any further than the occupational therapy literature. Human is a biological term that has no specific meaning for occupational therapists. Science is 'the product of a collective human enterprise to which scientists make individual contributions which are purified and extended by mutual criticism and intellectual co-operation' (Ziman 1978, quoted in Bench 1989, p. 149). The term has not been given a different meaning by occupational therapists.

Words can be used in a narrow, scientific sense to convey a precise meaning, as when the term 'micron' is used to signify an exact, small measurement. They can also be used in a poetic sense to convey shifting layers of meanings that depend as much on the perception and compre-hension of the listener as on the intention of the speaker. For example, do people have a precise, scientific understanding of the term 'nurse'? The word conjures up in most people's minds a variety of images, many of them glamorous. Most people would say confidently that they know what a nurse is, and yet their romantic vision is far removed from the current reality. Occupational therapy should perhaps be seeking to convey a more poetic understanding of its meaning and function, rather than an exact understanding.

Meanings are not fixed for all time but are temporarily fixed by the dominant group in a particular community at any one time, such as medicine or psychology in the field of health care. There is always the potential for another group to challenge the status quo. So far, occupa-tional therapists have failed either to create a new language to describe what we do or to change the meaning of the words we use.

Explaining occupational therapy

When occupational therapists are asked 'What do you do?' they tend to have difficulty finding a satisfactory answer. Madden (1984) recorded the explanations that new occupational therapy staff and students gave of the occupational therapy department and its therapeutic possibilities within a psychiatric unit, as though to patients and other professionals. She found that, with very few exceptions, the concepts of occupational therapy were explained extremely badly. The main problems were jargon, repetition and vagueness. She concluded that:

> After considering our taped explanations, it is easy to see that a listener may be no wiser for hearing them, and certainly no more likely to view psychiatric occupational therapy as making a signifi-cant and realistic contribution to treatment.

Lycett (1991) interviewed 46 occupational therapists employed in health or social services in Dorset to find out how they defined occupational therapy. She also asked interviewees how they felt about explaining occupational therapy. Sixty-seven percent of the therapists reported that they found it difficult to explain occupational therapy, and about 60 percent of these felt that the difficulty lay with the nature of the work or with other people's lack of understanding. The remaining 40 percent felt the problem was their own. Lycett found that there was no common approach to explaining occupational therapy among her subjects. A large variety of words and phrases were used so that most were only used by one person. The most frequently used words, such as independence and rehabilitation, did not differentiate occupational therapy from other health care professions.

In 1992, Beynon discussed the importance of giving information about occupational therapy to new clients in order to increase their motivation to participate in treatment. Beynon (p. 186) acknowledged that 'The language of occupational therapy differs from that used by other professional groups within the health service and will probably convey little meaning to the patient.' She suggested that explanations of occupational therapy should be graded to the individual's level of understanding and that different ways of providing information should be used, including writing down the aims of particular sessions.

The nature of what occupational therapists do does not translate easily into language. Much of their work is concerned with carrying out the tasks and activities of everyday life. Theories have been developed to define, categorise and explain the relationship between such concepts as skills, tasks, activities and occupations and these theories can be communicated verbally. However, the actual tasks and skills that occupational therapists work with are not so easy to put into words. For example, if a client needs to learn a new way of getting dressed after a stroke the therapist will demonstrate the new method and perhaps use physical and verbal prompts while the individual practises. It would be neither efficient nor effective to try to translate the whole process into words.

Another reason for difficulties occupational therapists have with saying what they do might be the breadth and variety of practice. Occupational therapy covers a broad range of fields, works with many problems, incorporates a wide spectrum of theories and a huge number of techniques and is concerned with complexity and individual difference. Language, particularly scientific language, cannot encompass the multiplicity and heterogeneity of occupational therapy practice.

Occupational therapy practice is client-centred rather than technique or skill centred. What the occupational therapist does on a particular occasion, with a particular client, is strongly influenced by factors in the immediate situation. Jenkins and Brotherton (1995, p. 332) wrote that: 'occupational therapy has a pragmatic orientation and rests on contact and first-hand experiences with clients and their worlds. It is indisputably client focused.' This means that what the occupational therapist does evolves in the context of the intervention and is not predetermined. It is easier for the therapist to say what she did in a particular case than to say in advance what she will do or to say in general terms what she does.

Why can't occupational therapists say what they do?

The precise nature of the difficulties that occupational therapists have with language has been clarified but the reasons for them have not yet been uncovered. This section looks at how language is used to convey meaning and the importance of power relationships in creating shared meanings. It then explores the position of occupational therapists in the fields in which they work and considers how they might be disadvantaged. The section ends with a discussion of the relationship between language and identity.

Misunderstanding occupational therapy

In order to understand why no satisfactory definition of occupational therapy has been agreed on, it is necessary to consider both the nature of language and the position of occupational therapy within the fields of health and social care.

The *Concise Oxford Dictionary* defined language as 'a vocabulary and way of using it prevalent in one or more countries'. This definition raises an important point about language: that it is used. A language, such as English, consists of a system of written and spoken words, grammar and pronunciation that, in use by particular individuals, will change in both form and meaning. That is, we can distinguish between language as an abstract system and the written or spoken performance of individuals.

Saussure (1974), a Swiss linguist, described language as a system of signs. Signs are made up of two aspects: the meaning or concept being referred to, which Saussure called the 'signified'; and the sound image or marks on a flat surface used to refer to the concept, called the 'signifier'. The term 'occupational therapy' is a linguistic sign that consists of the two words of the signifier and the meaning that these words convey, the signified. The meaning of signs is not intrinsic – that is, there is not necessarily any natural connection between a sign and the concept it signifies. 'Words themselves do not inherently contain meaning but depend upon a material context and a conscious subject to invest them with meaning' (Franklin 1985).

In order for language to be used for communication there has to be agreement between the speaker and listener on the meaning of the signifier within the context of that particular interaction. This meaning comes from:

- the intentions of the speaker;
- agreement about the meaning of words within the community that speaks the language being used (how words are defined in dictionaries, for example);
- the context in which the communication is taking place; and
- the perceptions and understanding of the listener.

The English language is in continuous use and changes all the time through use, albeit slowly. New words come into the language to signify new concepts or to signify old ones in a new way. Old, long-disused words come back into use with their original meanings, or with new ones. The meaning of commonly used words changes and evolves. Concepts change and evolve so that the words used to communicate them may no longer be adequate to convey their full meaning. There is a dynamic relationship between signifier and signified in which the two influence and modify each other.

Polatajko (1992) called the process of finding names for concepts 'naming', and the process of sharing meaning 'framing'. 'Naming is the act of giving a name to. Framing is organizing or schematizing experience...designed to share memory and understanding within a culture' (pp. 191–2).

Dickoff and James (1968) suggested that identifying and giving names to factors in a situation is the first level of theory development. 'The essential function of naming is the giving of a tag to enable reference back to, or the pointing to, or communicating about the factor conceived as having the name assigned. For a factor to have a name is for that factor to become mentionable' (p. 420). Polatajko (1992) claimed that 'Communication is based on the clear, precise sharing of meaning with another' and that 'what is important is the meaning a name holds' (p. 191).

In order to communicate effectively there must be a shared understanding of the meaning of names. First, the person communicating must find names for the concepts she wishes to communicate. Franklin (1985) wrote of the effect that finding words, or names, for things, can have: 'These words that may give us the means to say what we have always known but never known we knew can alter our relation to the world and to ourselves' (p. 5).

Secondly the communicator must find a way of giving names the meaning that she wishes to convey. Polatajko (1992, p. 191) wrote that:

> In occupational therapy we must determine the meaning we want to convey, consider the meaning our terms hold for others and then name or rename accordingly. Having done that we must work to have our meaning shared by others.

Our understanding of words comes from what they are not as much as from what they are. Saussure (1974) pointed out that language speakers are able to distinguish significant differences between sounds such as 't' and 'd' and it is these differences that enable different meanings to be given to each word. For example, 'tin' has a different meaning from 'din'. The concept of significant difference also applies to meanings. Levi-Strauss (1958), an anthropologist, introduced the concept of binary opposition to refer to systems of difference organised around binary opposite terms such as male–female, black–white or up–down.

Meanings are created out of difference. Our understanding of what something is comes partly out of what it is not, therefore the stronger the binary opposition the clearer the meaning should become (Franklin 1985).

Does the term occupational therapy convey a meaning strongly different from other terms? The *Concise Oxford Dictionary* defined physician as 'one who practises the healing arts including medicine and surgery'. It defined therapy as 'medical treatment of disease'. From their names, there is no clear and obvious difference between what a physician does and what an occupational therapist does, since what is communicated is that the purpose of both is to try to heal disease. Du Toit (1979) pointed out that in any language therapy is normally translated to mean treatment. 'TREATMENT immediately brings to mind synonyms such as to remedy, to doctor, to cure, to restore, which in turn has a strong medical association' (p. 429).

We also share the name therapy with several other professions, such as physiotherapy, speech and language therapy and art therapy. It is therefore necessary for the other word in our title, occupational, to make clear the difference. Occupation has been defined by the *Concise Oxford Dictionary* as 'what occupies one, means of passing one's time, temporary or regular employment, business, calling, pursuit' . In general usage the noun 'occupation' tends to be used to refer to a person's main job, whether paid or unpaid. The verb 'occupy' usually means keeping busy – hence, perhaps, the persistence of the idea that occupational therapists keep people busy (with craftwork). The adjective occupational is strongly associated with employment or work. For example, occupational health is the branch of healthcare concerned with occupational disease and injury – that is, health problems incurred at, or because of, work. In the public mind there is frequently confusion between occupational therapy and occupational health. All occupational therapy departments, whether in hospitals or academic institutions, are accustomed to having telephone calls and post put through to them that were intended for the occupational health department. So the name of the profession does not convey our difference.

Meanings are not fixed for all time but are temporarily fixed by the dominant group in a particular community at any one time, such as medicine or psychology in the field of health care. There is always the potential for another group to challenge the status quo. The failure of occupational therapists to change the meaning of the words we use is, at least partly, because we operate within discursive fields in which our discourse does not carry equal weight with that of the dominant group – always men and usually medicine. There is, therefore, an issue of power in the difficulty occupational therapists have in establishing their own knowledge base through creating a language of our own.

Knowledge, power and language

The concept of discursive fields was described by the French philosopher, Foucault (1970). These are ways of structuring social institutions and processes and of giving meaning to the world. Most of them are shaped and directed by men. Examples of discursive fields are the political system, the family, the education system and the law. Occupational therapists work within discursive fields that are strongly dominated by men, usually the field of medicine, although an increasing number in the UK are working within the field of law. So, in trying to have their voices heard, occupational therapists are doubly disadvantaged, as women and as non-doctors or non-lawyers. However, Weedon (1987) pointed out that the dominant discourses are sites of contest and are under constant challenge from alternative discourses. The dominant group attempts to retain and confirm its status by 'failing to recognize the knowledge and skills of those who might challenge their position as legitimate' (Richters 1991, p. 141).

Many therapists will have had the experience, in a ward round, of listening to the opinions of the medical staff on a particular patient and thinking that their own picture of this person is quite different. They may feel intimidated into not expressing what they have observed, or try to speak but not manage to be listened to, or give their professional opinion and have it ignored, or persist until their voice is heard. The opinion of a young, female therapist is unlikely to be accorded equal respect with that of more dominant, more senior or male members of the team. The doctor's truth is given more weight than the occupational therapist's truth. Many post-modern writers (for example Foucault 1970, Moors 1991) have claimed that knowledge is the outcome of a discourse through which a group of people gains the power to decide what is true and right and imposes that view on others. The occupational therapist might see a client's problem differently from the way the doctor sees it, but it is unlikely that her truth will be accepted above his because the discourse within the multidisciplinary healthcare team maintains the doctor in the dominant position. This dominance causes the nature of medical knowledge to be valued above the nature of occupational therapy knowledge. The dominant group in any discourse wins the authority to define problems and solutions.

Knowledge, as defined by Enlightenment thought, maintains its privileged status through four discourses.

- The agency of speech in establishing what is true
- The devaluing and exclusion of women's knowledge
- The valorisation of abstract knowledge over contextual knowledge
- The quest for a unitary truth

The agency of speech in establishing what is true

Different values are given to speech and writing. Derrida (cited by Sarup 1988) contended that, in the West, speech is privileged over written language, a priority which he called 'phonocentrism'. The spoken word is thought to carry an immediacy or presence that is lacking in the written text where meaning is always mediated by other factors such as time and distance. Phonocentrism can be seen in the culture of health care institutions where the ward round and the verbal pronouncements of medical staff still carry great weight in influencing patient management. It is as though the results of tests and assessments recorded in written reports have to be ratified by being spoken by the doctor.

In this verbal culture, women are disadvantaged. Hekman (1990), drawing on the work of the cultural linguist Walter Ong, suggested that the roots of Western academicism are both oral and agonistic. The purpose of agonistic activity is to have one truth accepted over another truth. This is a tradition that can be traced back to the ancient Greek custom of disputation. Oral disputation is inherently adversarial. Tannen (1992) claimed that men use conversations as opportunities to engage in verbal conflict in order to establish or display their status, whereas women converse in order to negotiate connections and reach consensus. Since men are the dominant group, male conversational styles are valued more highly than women's and women are seen as less effective disputants than men, rather than men being seen as less effective negotiators than women.

The devaluing and exclusion of women's knowledge

The Greek custom of disputation was carried through into the middle ages when knowledge was defined through verbal contests. Women were excluded from the production of knowledge because the language of disputation was Latin and most women did not learn Latin, therefore linguistic practices in the institutions that create knowledge (that is, have the power to state what is true) have always been structured along gendered lines. Hawkesworth (1989, p. 539, Balbus 1982, Bordo 1986, Ferguson 1985, citing Harding 1986 and Keller 1984) argued that knowledge itself is gendered:

> It is said that rationality, a tough, rigorous, impersonal, competitive, unemotional, objectifying stance, 'is inextricably intertwined with issues of men's gender identities' such as obsession with separation and individuation. It is said that 'distinctively (Western) masculine desires are satisfied by the preoccupation with method, rule and law-governed behavior and activity.' It is said that the

connections between masculinization, reification, and objectifica-
tion are such that should women attempt to enter the male realm
of objectivity, they have only one option: to deny their female
nature and adopt the male mode of being.

Belenky and colleagues (1986) carried out a study of women's thinking
from which they concluded that:

> conceptions of knowledge and truth that are accepted and articu-
> lated today have been shaped throughout history by the male-
> dominated majority culture. Drawing on their own perspectives
> and visions, men have constructed the prevailing theories, written
> history, and set values that have become the guiding principles for
> men and women alike. Our major educational institutions –
> particularly our secondary and postsecondary schools – were
> originally founded by men for the education of men . . . Relatively
> little attention has been given to modes of learning, knowing, and
> valuing that may be specific to, or at least common in, women. It is
> likely that the commonly accepted stereotype of women's
> thinking as emotional, intuitive, and personalized has contributed
> to the devaluation of women's minds and contributions, particu-
> larly in Western technologically oriented cultures, which value
> rationalism and objectivity. (p. 5)

This privileging of masculine ways of thinking means that, if women think
differently, their knowledge will be devalued, seen as deviant and
accorded lower status. Rationality, logic, objectivity and science are the
concepts usually associated with men's styles of thinking, whereas women
are seen as irrational, intuitive, subjective and artistic. Hekman (1990)
argued that, in Enlightenment thought, rationalism is the realm of the
knowing subject and only subjects can constitute knowledge. Since men
are defined as subjects and women as objects, women are defined as
incapable of producing knowledge and are excluded from intellectual life.

In order to make their voices heard within the multidisciplinary
health care team, occupational therapists find themselves having to
avoid describing patients in non-scientific terms such as 'She can't make
a cup of tea independently.' They may either apply standardised tests to
obtain a numerical score for what they have observed or dress up the
patient's functional level in 'scientific' language: 'Mrs Brown has the
physical and cognitive skills necessary to carry out simple tasks, but she
is unable to build them effectively into the complex sequences required
for function in daily life activities.'

Richters (1991, p. 123) described reason and rationality as 'highly
pretentious and pernicious forms of moral imperialism' through which
alternative modes of thinking are marginalised.

The valorisation of abstract knowledge over contextual knowledge

Enlightenment thought privileges an abstract rationality so that objective knowledge, which is said to exist independent of any particular context, is seen as more valid or more true than knowledge embedded in an individual situation. The process of producing scientific knowledge involves removing the social and historical circumstances on which the construction of the knowledge depended, so that accepted 'facts' come to be seen as existing independently of scientific endeavour. They are seen not as the constructions of the scientific process but as its discoveries. Latour and Woolgar (1980), in their study of laboratory life, demonstrated how a statement becomes a fact when it moves beyond the scope of sociological and historical explanation. Scientific knowledge is abstract knowledge.

A patient's problems are constituted through the discourse of institutional health care systems as expressed by the deliberations of the multidisciplinary team. A scientific approach to knowing what is wrong with a patient involves carrying out scientific tests, making objective observations and fitting the patient into an abstract framework which exists independently of his situation, such as the World Health Organisation International Classification of Diseases (ICD-10 1992). Jenkins (1994) described how the process of diagnosis rests on abstract principles and is detached from the patient's life context: 'its focus is . . . classificatory not relational or relativistic. Particularistic considerations, that is individual circumstances and possible mitigating contexts, are disregarded.' The patient is then labelled with a diagnosis that can be confirmed by further tests and observations.

The occupational therapist's approach, in contrast, 'does not revolve around abstract principles but on real life situations' (Jenkins and Brotherton 1995, p. 332). The patient's problem is framed by interaction between the patient and therapist in a process in which 'clients and practitioners learn together through repeated exposure to real world situations' (p. 335). This is not a scientific process, and the knowledge produced may not be testable by scientific methods, therefore it will be considered to have less validity than the medical diagnosis, irrespective of the relative use to the patient of the doctor's diagnosis and the occupational therapist's functional assessment. The dominant discourse is the one that refers back to abstract principles or knowledge.

The quest for a unitary truth

In Enlightenment thought, truth is unitary and multiple or competing explanations are not tolerated. In any one situation there is a single truth to be told. Western scientific endeavour is directed towards discovering the single truth about how the universe is organised and this has become a metaphor for Western philosophy, which engages in linear arguments that culminate in discovery of the ultimate truth.

The French philosopher, Irigaray (1977), linked the search for the one truth with the male anatomy, suggesting that the criteria for what is valid are based on the singularity and visibility of the erect penis:

> Truth must be, to start with, singular, unified, visible and whole if it is to stand up to scrutiny. The criteria for what is true, what is definitive, what holds up as evidence or has the status of the ontologically valid are the criteria of specularisability and discrete form. (Franklin 1985, pp. 13–14)

Hawkesworth (1989, p. 540) described reason as 'morphologically and functionally analogous to the male sex organ, linear, hard, penetrating but impenetrable'. She suggested that the privileging of evidence based on observation derives from men's need to 'valorize their own visible genitals against the threat of castration posed by women's genitalia'.

Western medicine subscribes to the metanarrative of progress towards a full understanding of the world and, in particular, of the nature of health and disease. When the truth has been discovered, medical science will triumph and disease will be eradicated. The doctor is the expert who holds the knowledge to control disease and cure the patient.

Occupational therapists, on the other hand, work with people who have chronic illness or permanent disability and are therefore concerned with the meaning that such illness or disability has for the individual rather than with understanding disease and effecting a cure. They aim to make small but significant changes in the lives of their clients in order to help them develop a sense of being able to manage better. The therapist's role is to help the patient to become his own expert.

Within healthcare settings acute, curative medicine is valued more highly than the alleviative function of occupational therapy because medicine is part of Enlightenment progress whereas occupational therapy is firmly located in the here and now.

Occupational therapists are in a trap. In order to be accepted as a full profession, with the benefits that this brings, of self-regulation and self-definition, occupational therapy must be able to show how it is different from other healthcare groups. If we fail to demonstrate our difference we cannot justify our existence as a separate profession in the competitive world of healthcare. If we succeed in being seen as different we will concomitantly be seen as inferior to the profession of medicine, because medicine holds the dominant position in Western healthcare and 'different from' equals 'inferior to'.

Creating identity through language

The concepts of difference and inferiority are embedded in Western language in binary opposition that always benefits one group over another. 'The role of systems of difference in the process of constructing meaning has been seen by many feminists as the basic process in patriarchy responsible for the polarization of sexual difference that ensures female inferiority' (Franklin 1985, p. 8). The difference between opposites allows for categorisation as good–bad, superior–inferior or dominant–subordinate. This means that the dominant group, in this case doctors, is the defining group and every different group is 'other' and, by implication, both inferior and subordinate. Occupational therapy, as a mainly female and characteristically feminine profession, is doubly inferior in relation to medicine which, although it is no longer primarily a male profession, remains masculine in nature. The male–female opposition is seen by many feminists as the fundamental form of opposition, more basic even than race or class (Weedon 1987).

This perception of inferiority is not only in the views that others have of occupational therapy but is also part of our identity as occupational therapists, because the language that others use to refer to us, and the language we use about ourselves, is important in creating our identity.

'Words are not simply static forms that are assigned to various external objects and ideas so as to convey the "real" meaning of the "real" world – far less to control (name) it or define its truths. "Reality" depends on one's point of view, and words are the basic building blocks we use to construct ourselves in relation to our world' (Franklin 1985, p. 2).

Occupational therapists are aware of the power of language. Bell (1991, p. 129) said that: 'The way we communicate to clients, peers, students, colleagues and the community at large . . . says much about the value we place on ourselves.' Webb (1990, p. 414) wrote of the adoption of the terminology of the marketplace by health services and asked:

> Why have we failed to notice that we are adopting more than just the language? It seems we have been anaesthetised in order to have our philosophy surgically removed and a donor philosophy implanted. And this donor philosophy is not about care, patients or people, but about . . . money.

We internalise the meanings that language gives us and the more we define ourselves as different the worse we feel about ourselves. This is because of a feature of people's understanding of themselves that post-structuralist theorists call 'subjectivity'. Our sense of self and ways of understanding the world and our relationship to it are not fixed, unique and coherent. 'Poststructuralism proposes a subjectivity which is precarious, contradictory and in process, constantly being reconstituted in discourse each time we think or speak' (Weedon 1987, p. 33). So, occupational therapists talking to other occupational therapists, or thinking about their own work, may feel comfortable with their identity, but as soon as they begin to interact with other professionals they are faced with alternative understandings of their role. They have become the subject of conflicting discourses. The result is often feelings of frustration, dissonance and dissatisfaction.

Occupational therapists are mostly women, but whether we work in clinical or academic settings we work in masculine environments. The professional and managerial structures within which we operate have been designed to allow for the expression and expansion of so-called male characteristics, interests and values: 'power, control and possession' (Cracknell 1989, p. 387). These qualities are reflected in the way that men use language. Feminist theorists claim that language itself is male defined 'and thus inevitably both constrains women's speech and reinforces male realities and male truths' (Franklin 1985, p. 2). The style of women's talk has been shown to differ from men's talk. Women's talk is hesitant, qualified and question-posing (Belenky et al. 1986), in contrast with men's need to 'fix, structure and codify' (Cracknell 1989, p. 387). Tannen (1992) described men's conversations as 'negotiations in which people try to achieve and maintain the upper hand, if they can, and to protect themselves from others' attempts to put them down' (p. 24). Women's conversations, on the other hand, are 'negotiations for closeness in which people try to seek and give confirmation and support, and to reach consensus' (op. cit. p. 25). The male style is seen as normative and, as the subordinate group, women, are seen to depart from the norm. As a result of this, women's communications are typically not valued as highly as men's, either by men or by women. Women talk less than men in mixed groups and are more likely to be interrupted (Belenky et al. 1985). Both these points make it very difficult for the occupational therapist to be heard and she may begin to accept the view that what she knows is not worth saying.

Power and control within the system of healthcare are held by the medical profession and all other professionals are subordinate to the physician (Friedson 1970). Occupational therapists are not only trying to make themselves heard using androcentric language, but they are trying to be heard by a dominant profession which uses language to reinforce its own realities and truths. Lugones and Spelman (1983, p. 575) gave a powerful description of Hispanic women's experience of trying to communicate with non-Hispanic women. This passage captures something of the feeling that occupational therapists experience within their work settings.

We and you do not talk the same language. When we talk to you we use your language: the language of your experience and your theories. We try to use it to communicate our world of experience. But since your language and your theories are inadequate in expressing our experiences, we only succeed in communicating our experience of exclusion. We cannot talk to you in our language because you do not understand it. So the brute facts that we understand your language and that the place where most theorising . . . is taking place is your place, both combine to require that we either use your language and distort our experience. . . or that we remain silent.

Conclusion

There are both risks and opportunities for occupational therapists as we approach the end of the twentieth century. To what extent are these minimised or exaggerated by the difficulties we have in communication?

If occupational therapists cannot say what they are and what they do, they remain vulnerable to having their role and function defined by others. In the past, doctors have told the occupational therapist what to do. Now, it is likely to be general managers or accountants who decide what are the most cost-effective and efficient modes of service delivery. If we cannot say what we do, we cannot measure our effectiveness in ways that reflect the true nature of the work and may find that others measure what is easily measurable and ignore the less visible aspects of occupational therapy.

Occupational therapists run the risk of losing what little status and autonomy they have managed to win during this century. They risk having goals imposed on them that have nothing to do with individual clients or enablement but are about clearing beds and creating a fast turnover. The flexibility that is such a strong feature of the occupational therapy approach will be lost as the therapist tries to meet the requirements of contracts and predesigned procedures. Words set boundaries to keep others out but they also constrain what we do, and if others say those words then the occupational therapist has lost her autonomy.

The concepts of generic therapy and multiskilling should not pose any threats to occupational therapists, who are traditionally willing to use any techniques that work for the client, with the proviso that they are not invasive or against the individual's wishes. However, if managers determine the range of skills that each profession should adopt, occupational therapists may be left feeling even less clear about what is unique about their practice. This may be the factor that has enabled the profession to retain its feminine characteristics. Alleviative medicine is not concerned with cure, or progress towards cure. It is concerned with quality of life and enablement.

The features of occupational therapy that seem to make the profession weak are the same features that are its strengths. Occupational therapists are not experts, they do not know what is best for their clients. The philosophy underpinning practice is that each person has the capacity to know what he wants and to work towards it. Occupational therapy is concerned with enabling clients to take control of their own lives, or aspects of their own lives. It is concerned with individual lives, abilities, aspirations and truths. The occupational therapist focuses on practical issues and works with each client within specific contexts to determine the best course of action for that person at that time.

Does it matter that occupational therapists cannot say what they do? The profession has survived by being useful, not by being powerful. There are dangers to occupational therapists in the world of contracts, predetermined protocols for intervention and measurable outcomes, which may take away some of the flexibility and responsiveness that make the profession useful but there will always be a need for someone to work with the little activities of everyday life with people who have problems of function.

References

Barris R (1984) Towards an image of one's own: sources of variation in the role of occupational therapists in psychosocial practice. Occupational Therapy Journal of Research 4(1): 3–23.

Belenky MF, Clinchy BM, Goldberger NR and Tarule JM (1986) Women's Ways of Knowing: the Development of Self, Voice and Mind. New York: Basic.

Bell J (1991) Sylvia Docker lecture: communicating a professional image. Australian Occupational Therapy Journal 38(3): 127–35.

Bench RJ (1989) Health science, natural science and clinical knowledge. Journal of Medicine and Philosophy 14: 147–64.

Beynon S (1992) Stranger in a strange land: a consumer guide to occupational therapy. British Journal of Occupational Therapy 55(5): 186–8.

Blom-Cooper L (1989) Occupational Therapy: an Emerging Profession in Health Care. London: Duckworth.

Breines EB (1984) An attempt to define purposeful activity. American Journal of Occupational Therapy 38(8): 543–4.

Breines EB (1995) Understanding 'occupation' as the founders did. British Journal of Occupational Therapy 58(11): 458–60.

Busuttil J (1992) Psychosocial occupational therapy: from myth and misconception to multidisciplinary team member. British Journal of Occupational Therapy 55(12): 457–61.

Clark PN (1979) Human development through occupation: theoretical frameworks in contemporary occcupational therapy practice, Part 1. American Journal of Occupational Therapy 33(8): 505–14.

Clark FA, Parham D, Carlson ME, Frank G, Jackson J, Pierce D, Wolfe RJ, Zemke R (1991) Occupational science: academic innovation in the service of occupational therapy's future. American Journal of Occupational Therapy 45(4): 300–10.

Cracknell E (1989) Conflicts for the female therapist: some reflections. British Journal of Occupational Therapy 52(10): 386–8.

Dickoff J, James P (1968) A theory of theories: a position paper. Nursing Research 17(1): 197–203.

Drever J (1952) A Dictionary of Psychology. Harmondsworth: Penguin.

Dunkin EN, Goble RA (1982) Nursing and occupational therapy: focus for the future. British Journal of Occupational Therapy 45(2): 45–8.

Du Toit E (1979) A definition of occupational therapy for occupational therapists. Proceedings of the Seventh International Congress of the World Federation of Occupational Therapists. Jerusalem, WFOT.

Engelhardt HT (1977) Definitive occupational therapy: the meaning of therapy and the virtues of occupation. American Journal of Occupational Therapy 31(10): 666–72.

Foucault M (1970) (trans. Sheridan A) The Order of Things: an Archeology of the Human Sciences. New York: Pantheon.

Franklin S (1985) Luce Irigaray and the Feminist Critique of Language. University of Kent at Canterbury Women's Studies Occasional Papers No. 6.

Friedson E (1970) The Profession of Medicine. New York: Dodd Mead.

Green M (1977) Development or oblivion? British Journal of Occupational Therapy 51(3): 78–80.

Green S (1991) Shaking our foundations, Part 2. Into the future. British Journal of Occupational Therapy 54(2): 53–6.

Hagedorn R (1995) Occupational Therapy: Perspectives and Processes. Edinburgh: Churchill Livingstone.

Hall M (1989) New dissertation available on loan. British Journal of Occupational Therapy 52(6): 254.

Hawkesworth ME (1989) Knowers, knowing, known: feminist theory and claims of truth. Signs Journal of Women in Culture and Society 4(31): 533–57.

Hekman SJ (1990) Gender and Knowledge: Elements of a Postmodern Feminism. Cambridge: Polity.

Hollis V (1993) Core skills and competencies: Part 1, what is experience? British Journal of Occupational Therapy 56(2): 48–50.

Horner S (1983) Letter to the editor. British Journal of Occupational Therapy 46(8): 237.

Irigaray L (1977) Women's exile. Ideology and Consciousness 1.

Jenkins M (1994) Occupational Therapy: Perspectives on the Effectiveness of Practice. Thesis submitted to the University of Ulster for the degree of PhD.

Jenkins M, Brotherton C (1995) In search of a theoretical framework for practice, part 2. British Journal of Occupational Therapy 58(8): 332–6.

Katz N, Sachs D (1991) Meaning ascribed to major professional concepts: a comparison of occupational therapy students and practitioners in the United States and Israel. American Journal of Occupational Therapy 45(2): 137–45.

Kielhofner G, Burke JP (1980) A model of human occupation, part 1: conceptual framework and content. American Journal of Occupational Therapy 34(9): 572–81.

Latour B, Woolgar S (1979) Laboratory Life: the Social Construction of Scientific Facts. Beverley Hills: Sage.

Levi-Strauss C (1958/1972) (trans. Jacobson C and Schoeff BG) Structural Anthropology. Harmondsworth: Penguin.

Lugones M, Spelman V (1983) Have we got a theory for you! Feminist theorem cultural imperialism and the demand for 'the women's voice'. Women's Studies International Forum 6(6): 573–81.

Lycett R (1991) What is occupational therapy? An examination of the definitions given by occupational therapists. British Journal of Occupational Therapy 54(11): 411–14.

MacDonald K (1990) Letter to the editor. British Journal of Occupational Therapy 53(8): 341.

Madden A (1984) Explaining psychiatric occupational therapy: an art in itself? British Journal of Occupational Therapy 47(1): 15–17.

Mocellin G (1988) A perspective on the principles and practice of occupational therapy. British Journal of Occupational Therapy 51(1): 4–7.

Moncur A (1994) A terrible cloth to bear. Guardian, 5 September.

Moors A (1991) Women and the orient. In Nencel L, Pels P (eds) Constructing Knowledge: Authority and Critique in Social Science. London: Sage.

Mosey AC (1985) Eleanor Clarke Slagle lecture, 1985: A monistic or a pluralistic approach to professional identity? American Journal of Occupational Therapy 39(8): 504–9.

Mosey AC (1986) Psychosocial components of occupational therapy. New York: Raven Press.

Nelson DL (1988) Occupation: form and performance. American Journal of Occupational Therapy 42(10): 633–41.

Polatajko HJ (1992) Naming and framing occupational therapy: a lecture dedicated to the life of Nancy B. Canadian Journal of Occupational Therapy 59(4): 189–99.

Reed KL, Sanderson SN (1980) Concepts of occupational therapy. Baltimore, MD: Williams & Wilkins.

Reilly M (1962) Occupational therapy can be one of the great ideas of 20th century medicine. American Journal of Occupational Therapy 16(1): 1–9.

Reilly M (1969) The educational process. American Journal of Occupational Therapy 23(4): 299–307.

Richters A (1991) Fighting symbols and structures: postmodernism, feminism and women's health. In Nencel L, Pels P (eds) Constructing Knowledge: Authority and Critique in Social Science. London: Sage.

Sachs D and Jarus T (1992) Dimensions Affecting Occupational Therapists' Definition of the Profession. Poster presentation. Hong Kong International Occupational Therapy Conference.

Sarup M (1988) An Introductory Guide to Post-Structuralism and Postmodernism. New York: Harvester Wheatsheaf.

Saussure F de (1974) A Course in General Linguistics. London: Fontana.

Schön D (1983) The Reflective Practitioner: How Professionals Think in Action. New York: Basic.

Shannon PD (1977) The derailment of occupational therapy. American Journal of Occupational Therapy 31(4): 229–34.

Sheik AJ, Boultan D (1992) Why occupational therapy? Psychiatric Bulletin 16: 406–8.

Stewart A (1994) Empowerment and enablement: occupational therapy 2001. British Journal of Occupational Therapy 57(7): 248–54.

Tannen D (1992) You Just Don't Understand: Women and Men in Conversation. London: Virago.

Unsworth CA (1993) The concept of function. British Journal of Occupational Therapy 56(8): 287–92.

Webb C (1990) Nursing as a profession – towards a new model. University of Manchester, inaugural lecture.

Weedon C (1987) Feminist practice and poststructuralist theory. Cambridge: Blackwell.

Wilcock AA (1993) Biological and sociocultural aspects of occupation, health and health promotion. British Journal of Occupational Therapy 56(6): 200–3.

Woods A (1990a) Letter to the editor. British Journal of Occupational Therapy 53(11): 471.

Woods A (1990b) Letter to the editor. British Journal of Occupational Therapy 53(6): 248.

World Health Organisation (1992) The ICD-10 Classification of Mental and Behavioural Disorders: Clinical Descriptions and Diagnostic Guidelines. Geneva: World Health Organisation.

Yerxa EJ, Clark F, Jackson J, Pierce D, Stein C, Frank G, Parham D, Zemke R (1990) An introduction to occupational science, a foundation for occupational therapy in the 21st century. Occupational Therapy in Health Care 6(4): 1–17.

Yerxa EJ (1993) Occupational science: a new source of power for participants in occupational therapy. Occupational Science: Australia 1(1): 3–10.

Chapter 9
Oil and water

MARY PERKS

'Doing to' or 'being with'

'You ought to' and 'Why don't you?' are phrases that anyone who has undertaken counselling training will recognise as the kind of thing you are not supposed to say to a client. Such phrases seem to introduce advice, and counselling is not about advice giving but about enabling clients to make their own decisions. If someone seems to want advice, it is assumed they do not understand what counselling is, and this is explained, perhaps a little patronisingly. If the counsellor wants to make a suggestion or offer information, he or she must first take off the counsellor's hat by saying, 'I am not now in my counsellor's role, but . . .' The use of this formula, like the clapper board in film directing, is a concrete and observable indication of a change of roles, which is supposed to obviate the risk to the counsellor. It is almost a magic formula to protect the counsellor and, as such, bears some resemblance to obsessional ritual.

I am playing devil's advocate here. It is, of course, right that counselling should not be about giving advice, although an occasional blurring of boundaries and admittance of a foreign element, rather than being a threat to the process, might enhance it. An overstrict adherence to roles and preservation of boundaries can destroy the very thing they are designed to protect. The exclusion of outside elements can produce an inner impoverishment and prevent the free interplay of internal and external. I shall return to this point, as the relationship of internal and external is central to this chapter.

Both the origins of words and the images they evoke are revealing for the development of ideas and the contemplative element in counselling. The focus on the present moment, which renders 'You ought to' and 'Why don't you' inappropriate and jarring, is contained in the word itself. Counselling means 'sitting down with'. It comprises the idea of stillness, being relaxed while in a state of alert attention, and of relationship – being with a particular person. Attention and relationship are the ingredients of contemplation, which has connotations of prayer but which is also present in other kinds of experience. There are elements of exclusivity and particularity – the counsellor is concerned with that client alone at that moment – and of focusing on the present. And there is self-emptying in order to attend to the client at a deep level. Simone Weil (1973) writes:

> Attention consists of suspending our thought . . . our thought should be empty, waiting, not seeking anything, but ready to receive . . . the object which is to penetrate it . . . Those who are unhappy have no need for anything . . . but people capable of giving them their attention. The capacity to give one's attention to a sufferer is a very rare and difficult thing . . .
>
> In the first legend of the Grail, it is said that the Grail . . . belongs to the first comer who asks the guardian of the vessel, a king three-quarters paralysed by the most painful wound, 'What are you going through?'
>
> The love of our neighbour . . . simply means being able to say to him: 'What are you going through?'
>
> This way of looking is first of all attentive. The soul empties itself of all its own contents in order to receive into itself the being it is looking at, just as he is, in all his truth.

The French word 'attente' means both waiting and attention. Waiting, in English, usually has temporal connotations, being in expectation of a future event. More rarely, and especially in a religious context, it means attention, openness, receptivity. I have heard Simone Weil's idea of attention referred to as an advanced empathy, a term which, with its nuances of standard assessment and professionalism, somehow diminishes the quality of what she is describing, which is something more numinous, a human and spiritual process transcending assumed roles.

'You ought to' and 'Why don't you' are also the most common responses when you show someone your painting. I knew immediately what a friend meant when she said, 'Whatever you do, people always want you to do something else.' When I said to my father, who is a poet, 'I suppose people say "You ought to" and "Why don't you" even more with poetry than with art,' he gave a wry smile. Many people who have engaged in creative activity have encountered this response. It can be as jarring as the intrusion of advice into counselling. Immersed in your work, or in enjoying the finished picture, you are suddenly asked to look beyond it, to see it as part of a system, a point in progression towards a goal with possible commercial implications. The relationship between creator and created, like that between counsellor and client, is one of exclusivity and is akin to love. Again, there are religious parallels. The finished work takes on a kind of independence or life of its own. You sense it has always existed, that its appearance at this particular moment was not entirely within your control. You have been a channel for its creation of itself, just as the counsellor is a catalyst for the client's self-discovery. The exclusiveness of your feelings for it arises from the sense of its uniqueness, as of a mother for her child. Art therapy, being a bridge between counselling and art, brings together two forms of contemplation. There is attention and relationship between the counsellor and client and between counsellor and created object. Instead of a pair we have a triad, the counselling relationship taken a stage further into the realm of internal imagery made concrete. It can be as destructive for the therapist as for the counsellor to say of the image, 'You ought to' or 'Why don't you,' in relation either to development of the technique and possible public recognition or to action on the basis of its emotional content.

Similar issues arise when looking at work in the artist's absence, as in a gallery. You can stand before a painting, absorbing it into yourself, alone with the object of contemplation, shutting out for a moment other concerns. Or you can see the painting within the context of the artist's entire oeuvre, comparing it with earlier or later work, referring away from the painting itself. This difference can be seen among visitors to stately homes. Some enjoy the objects for themselves, delighting in their qualities and the atmosphere they evoke. Theirs is an internal, intuitive response to what they see. Others require facts. They are text-based sightseers, referring constantly to the guidebook, looking only where told to look. A possible third group is those who ask whether the family still lives there. Here, there is an element of predatory voyeurism, of ogling the rich, of taking a peep into an inaccessible world.

This same voyeurism is seen elsewhere. An artist working out of doors has an irresistible attraction. Society both fears and glorifies art, views it at once with suspicion and admiring envy. Onlookers make comments such as 'What's that technique called?' 'How long has it taken?' 'What are you going to do with it?' 'What's it for?' The first response refers away from the work to an external authority. You are using a named technique that someone else has taught you. The second places the work within a time framework. It is a point in an exterior process. There are inferences of career planning, and the phrase 'time is money' hovers in the wings. The last two remarks posit the notion of a finite goal, drawing attention away from the work to something outside and beyond. There is a diminishing of the work. It cannot simply exist for itself but must be for or about something else. There is displacement, a removal from the present situation to another, not yet realised.

A duality is now emerging, of which counselling and art are paradigms: the interior, intuitive and individual qualities of life, centred on being, and the external, categorising, collective elements of life, centred on doing. Now we explore how Western culture promotes the latter to the detriment of the former.

'Being' in an ego-dominated society

'You ought to', 'Why don't you?' 'What are you going to do with it?' 'What's it for?' have a mechanistic ring, conveying a sense of pivotal movement, of turning on a hinge or of cogs in a wheel, moving from A to B via C to achieve D. They are finite, suggesting linear progression within a time framework, referential in that they look away from the observed object to something beyond and subordinating, making the object a means to an end, not existing by itself and for itself.

The ubiquity and predictability of these responses reflect an agenda, a distinct undercurrent in Western culture. Our minds are channelled in such a way that such responses spring automatically to our lips. Our mindset is one of progression, of proactive looking forward, everything we undertake being *for* something else. We live in the future, always at one remove from the present. Each activity must fit a greater whole, not in an interior and holistic sense but in an external, systemic sense. It is part of your career, a means to material success. I call this attitude projectionist or progressionist thinking, or process philosophy. It is closely linked to the dominance of the external, proactive ego over the internal, contemplative id. Divisions between areas of the human psyche, between reason and fantasy or body, mind and spirit, have characterised Western philosophy and psychology. Freud (1964) coined the terms 'ego' and 'id' and psychiatry defined mental illness as breakdown of ego, the loss of external control. Western theology has also taken up this thinking. In some Eastern religions, notably Hinduism and Buddhism, contemplation, the attentive relationship between the individual and God, forms the mainspring of life. Action radiates from inner stillness, reflected in eastern cultures by their sense of interconnectedness and timelessness, the feeling that life is a circle rather than a straight line. Christianity began as an eastern religion. Drawing apart, going into the desert, climbing the mountain, being alone, were prominent features that have become lost or discarded in the course of its weaving into the fabric of ego-dominated culture. It is reduced to a legalistic system of dos and don'ts, reflecting the Western need for enumerative, finite measure, or is bolted onto life, prayer being a means to material goals rather than a relationship. The Christian doctrine of atonement, the idea of paying a penalty on behalf of another, has a transactional quality and suggests movement towards a goal, revealing the dominance of projectionist ego. But the root of the word *at-one-ment* suggests spirit rather than mechanism, being rather than doing, a self-emptying identification with suffering which is the nature of counselling and contemplation.

The suspicion with which creative activity is viewed arises from its identification with the unconscious id – that which cannot be boundaried or controlled. It becomes acceptable only when brought within the scope of projectionist values, as the feminine is acceptable only insofar as it imitates the masculine, or black culture is acceptable insofar as it copies the West. Healthcare institutions are microcosms of society, reflecting these trends. As an art therapist in the field of mental health, I asked a colleague why the art therapy service had never been expanded. She said, 'It's because when you walk by, all you see is people working on their own thing. Nothing's happening! Why not get them painting a mural? It would show we were dynamic, that we were really doing something. Unless we justify ourselves, we'll be closed down.'

I call this the Muriel Syndrome (although murals are just one example of what art therapists are often expected to organise) or being project bound, unable to value work unless it comes under a collective heading. The overall identity and external show inherent in a project fulfil the demands of projectionist thinking while being in antithesis to the interior, intuitive nature of art therapy. My colleague's remark contains the quality of fear that underlies projectionism and takes several forms. When encountering someone in distress, we feel helpless. We might make them a cup of tea, anything to give us something to do and remove us from the situation. This removal resembles the outward referencing of the question, 'What is it for?' which comes from not knowing what to say and needing to break the silence that is really the deepest acknowledgement of the other. There is a centrifugal movement, flight from the core reality that is that person or that object. The essence of art and counselling, however, is being with, willing to hold the distress or take the object into yourself. 'Don't just do something, sit there,' might be a client's cry, reversing the well-worn saying and the value system that places doing above being. We have an innate fear of finding ourselves in that space, the fear of silence being shown in the indiscriminate use of the radio as background noise, deadening thought and feeling.

We need not only 'do' but should observe ourselves doing, in order to prove our value to ourselves, to satisfy our inner projectionist voice. Otherwise, we experience existential anxiety. We are profoundly uncomfortable with silence, ambiguity and unfinishedness. We also need to justify ourselves to others, especially those above us. The result is an internal splitting, our attention being half on the job and half on how it is viewed by authority.

There is another kind of fear – that of the power inherent in individuality. I have witnessed devaluation, dismissal and even destruction of clients' work that does not form part of a project initiated by staff, having a corporate image and unified by an externally imposed, predetermined theme. Individuality is dangerous, possibly because it may signal the beginnings of real independence on the client's part, which is the last thing to be desired. The reaction against wholly self-conceptualised work is so instinctual and primitive that it seems to indicate some deep agenda. Paradoxically, the output of work in an art room is often prolific enough to satisfy the demand for production, but this is never acknowledged. Individual work is denied, it is invisible. Only projects count. This can occasion an ongoing trauma and hurt which the art therapist must struggle to contain. He or she may feel profoundly isolated, unable to share the inner vision and exhausted by the constant effort of swimming against the tide. It is culture shock in microcosm, a clash of unwritten philosophies creating a sense of alienation, of speaking a different language from your colleagues.

The need for goals towards which progress can be measured is an aspect of projectionism. Goal and purpose are synonyms but evoke contrasting imagery. Goal is surface, linear and finite, suggesting a track, a mechanical movement from A to B. Art therapy does not have a goal, but rather a purpose, a word expressing the inner meaning or spirit of a thing, evoking the image of a circle, a centre, a point of infinity or timeless present. It is an intuitive work, even numinous, expressing essence rather than outworking, and concerned with attention and relationship. These cannot be measured or proved at second hand but can only be experienced and known in the moment. Your self-justification, therefore, has to be within yourself. You have to bear the angst of authenticity.

'All you can do is dig your trench and stay there. If you raise your head above the ground you get shot at' – a colleague's comment about the NHS Trust, which employs us. This kind of battle imagery had also occurred to me. Projectionism has always been present but it seems to have intensified, creating a sense of the tightening of a screw or the speeding up of a film. The clamour for project-based work as self-justification resembles the building of fortifications. Staff dig ditches and drive in stakes, the 'Muriel' being a metaphorical wall of defence, a hedge against redundancy. Another image is of concentric circles, client contact forming the core, with layers of management spiralling out. Each level must justify itself to the next, creating a division in attention. As energy is directed increasingly outwards there is a centrifugal effect that creates an inner vacuum, an inner impoverishment leading to a frantic polishing of the exterior as compensation. It is a Christmas tree bauble, with a shiny outside but no substance or, to use a strikingly similar word, a Tower of Babel, an edifice of inauthenticity that compounds and pyramids upon itself. The internal destruction leads ultimately to the destruction of the exterior as it becomes more brittle. The tower becomes top-heavy and finally topples. I define authenticity as acting from the centre, having internal unity, not observing your actions or thinking how others might view them. I believe much unspoken depression within health service personnel is due to the sense of entrapment in an inauthentic system, whilst longing for deeper values.

A survey of attitudes

Ego culture is not of itself materialistic but is value-neutral. The ego attributes of reason and self-control were, to the Stoical philosophers, both the ultimate happiness and the ultimate good, but concepts have become wedded, in the West, to materialism. In other words, the actual content of projectionist thinking is accumulation and status, ego providing the bare bones on which the flesh of materialism is hung. The forward thrust of Western motivation is self-improvement within certain parameters. The projectionist ethos of mental health services, therefore, incorporates a health-success equation, an identification of health with a notion of advancement that has more in common with educative rather than with therapeutic processes. The sense of a more determined rallying behind the projectionist flag is broadly represented by a move from therapy to education, a trend most evident in mental health day care where recent dissociation from the institution of the hospital has produced a consolidation of identity and role.

To test this, I researched the attitudes of day care staff within an NHS Trust responsible for mental health services in a rural county. I conducted a number of structured interviews based on a confidential questionnaire, six with individuals and nine with groups, each interview lasting about 30 minutes. Participants were given the questionnaire at the beginning of the interview and invited to discuss it. They were asked, in addition, to fill in the questionnaire after the interview and return it if they wanted to. Participants included day centre staff, community mental health teams, hospital and social services managers overseeing day-care facilities and several clients. Thirty-two questionnaires were subsequently completed and returned. The quotations that follow are taken from either interviews or questionnaires.

Interviewees were asked to assess day centre activities, to identify omissions in services, pinpoint major changes and express their feelings about the Trust's values. The questionnaire was designed to allow flexibility in interpretation and response, an approach that created unease. I sometimes sensed bafflement and disorientation. The comment was heard, 'I wish it were multiple choice.' There was a need for enumeration, a flight into finite categories at the same time as a desire for and appreciation of the chance for individual expression. This ambivalence reflected that described earlier; a sense of being constrained by the system and wishing, in a way, to comply with it, coupled with a recognition of and desire for alternative values and approaches. Several respondents felt unable to comment on values without referring to the mission statement of the service, a text-based response similar to that of the second type of stately home visitor, the appeal to an outside authority in the form of something written down, rather than reliance on internal intuition or reference to the ways in which the service impinged on individuals personally. The frequency of this response took me by surprise since, in answering that question myself, it would not have occurred to me to refer to an official document. I realised that, in formulating the question, I had been unconsciously seeking an intuitive response and had not taken into account differences in personality. A minority did respond personally, for example:

> The Trust's values are well meaning but limited in vision. It appears business-orientated, it's become a numbers game, a shop window syndrome. Modern Trusts are driven by political doctrine and expediency. More emphasis is on public relations, looking as though you are doing a good job without this necessarily being the case. Whatever we feel, the reality is we must work with what we have.

Four major themes emerged from the data: preoccupation with the concept of normality, concern with the relationship between the day centre and society, emphasis on skills and reference to socialisation.

Normality

The phrase 'What is normal?' is a cliché, albeit based on the recognition that normality is indefinable, each individual being unique. Paradoxically, however, a strong emphasis on normality underlies mental health day care. The words 'normal', 'normality', 'normalising' and 'normalisation' constantly occurred in the study. For example:

> Mental health is being normal, having a good job and a good woman, coping. It is the ability to function adequately in a normal society, to do normal, everyday things. Activities should challenge the individual's concept of being not normal. There is now more emphasis on moving on and moving out.

'Functioning adequately' presupposes a specific point at which a person becomes adequate. Imagistically, there is vertical and horizontal movement, a sense of advancing through succeeding levels before sliding out at the top like a meal in a restaurant lift, a self-replenishing, conveyor-belt process. Normality is seen as being in opposition to institutionalisation, the move from hospital to day care a step towards real life or normality. The asylum, literally a place of retreat or the still centre of real life, was, and still is, seen as an alternative to real life, a place to which people went for whom real life was untenable, an alongside world with which there was no free commerce. Asylums in the Victorian era became societies in their own right, reflecting society outside. Treatment was interventionist, curative, having something done to you, the doctor–patient relationship paramount, with its unequal power balance. The concept of normalisation is seen as the breakdown of this duality, this divide:

> We should get away from the idea of care. Activities should reflect day-to-day living; integrate the individual into mainstream society. There is a move towards real world skills and education. There should be replication with what people do outside the service. Mental health is functioning out there in the real world.

Relationship with society

There is a sense of veering round, returning to the point where you began, like a boat putting out to sea, which describes a curve and returns to shore, or a missile appearing to move rapidly away from earth and then going into orbit. There appears a bifurcation of aims, some seeing the day centre as part of society – going into the community, using community facilities – others seeing it as a reflector of society. The use of the word 'replication' is intriguing. Used in genetics, it means the making of an exact copy. Integration implies free interplay; replication implies a divide – a mirror of life rather than part of it, a looking-glass world in which you rehearse for life. It is a return to the asylum in a different form although, whereas for many the asylum was a final desti-nation, the mirror world a permanent alternative to real life, the inten-tion in day care is that the rehearsal shall become the play. The integrative and replicatory functions of day care may not, therefore, be mutually exclusive, though there appears a duality of which interested professionals may be unaware.

An example of replication is the rehabilitation kitchen, a facility found in most day centres. Importance is attached to learning domestic skills as a stage towards independence. The kitchen is designed to resemble, as far as possible, the normal kitchen outside. But who decides what constitutes a normal kitchen and by what criteria? There is a sense of artificial creation, of building a stage set, of aping real life. Moreover, constructing a typical environment carries the danger of denial of individuality, a watering down and reduction to a characterless average. A patient I knew, who had spent some time in Broadmoor special hospital, was, on admission to the hospital, made to remove all but one of her five pairs of earrings. A normal person with such decoration might be regarded as eccentric but a patient must remain within tighter bound-aries of normality determined by the health care system. Just as a woman in a man's world must be better than a man, so a mental patient must be more normal than normal. The logical conclusion of normalisation is, therefore, a loss of individuality, erosion of those edges that make us human. The normal life, which is presumably the goal of normalisation, is founded on values that are both system determined and ego-material-istic. As one respondent said: 'Mental health is being confident, having a positive self-image. There is a focus on doing and achieving. Activities should give a sense of achievement . . . produce work that wins praise.'

Confidence and self-esteem are seen in terms of achievement based on activity rather than on a sense of intrinsic worth, inner peace independent of circumstance, identity that transcends conventional measures of success. This is the recognition of a spiritual dimension, not in a narrow religious sense, since we have seen how Western religion has espoused projectionist culture, but as a deep searching for internal rootedness and meaning. Although 'moving on and moving out', expressive of the integrative day centre function, suggest greater interplay between internal and external than does the concept of replication, they begin with the external, leaving an inner vacuum. Art therapy is little understood because it seeks to start in the space behind this starting point, and conceives of creativity as transcending conventional boundaries of art, concerning itself with attention and being, rather than with socio-artistic success. The dislocation between internal and external produces external fragmentation, as happens in schizophrenia, with increasing division into finite units. This is shown in the burgeoning bureaucracy within health services (a collective schizophrenia), the demand to break everything down into its component parts.

Emphasis on skills

The word 'skills', with its shortness, its plurality, conveys slickness, enumeration and empty brittleness. You become subliminally aware of its constant repetition, resembling hammer blows. After a while, it jars like a musical instrument which, when heard for too long on its own without the relief of other instruments, begins to hurt the ear:

> We need more work with problem-solving and social skills, more crafts – increase in motivation. There is more emphasis on domestic rehabilitation, social skills training, a move towards skill-based therapies. The philosophy is 'salvation is in education' or 'the devil makes work for idle hands'.

The institutionalisation from which normalisation represents a flight is still apparent but in disguised form. The word endings of normalisation and socialisation give them an interventionist ring, evoking a predetermined package – a fixed process to be followed; passive, subservient patients and active, powerful staff. 'People become commodities, to be moved through the system', was one comment. By substituting the words normalising and socialising, the emphasis changes. The process arises from within rather than being imposed from without; patients become self-directing and staff move into a position alongside rather than face-to-face. But there remains the assumption of normality as an absolute and a valid goal.

Socialisation

> We need groups which encourage interaction, interactional activities, social activities, socialising with others, being able to mix with other people. We don't do individualised work, we are group-based. Normal life is to be part of a group, so that is how we operate.

Both normalisation and socialisation suggest working from without. Socialisation sounds interventionist, socialising more spontaneous, but both suggest superficiality, an assumed bonhomie and an emphasis on numbers, the group being of greater value than one-to-one work. 'There's no-one here!' is the anxious cry when there are fewer clients present than usual, meaning 'We're not seen to be doing!' Two or three gathered together are of no account in worldly terms. Relationship conveys a different meaning. Relationship is to socialisation as purpose is to goal – one being of the essence, the other imposed. One interviewee commented, 'You have to be at ease within yourself before you can relate to others.' While partly agreeing, I feel this suggests that solitude is a stage on the way to relationship, the precursor and ground of relationship. But this is a false duality. What we perceive as solitude is really a form of relationship that, with attention, forms the equation of contemplation. One possible significance of the notion of a trinity, present in other religions as well as in Christianity, is that relatedness exists within the godhead itself, that we experience relationship because it already exists within God's nature. Creation, existence itself, is dependent on relationship. Relationship is our primary reality, therefore, no matter how far we penetrate the core of reality, we never leave relationship behind or pass on to aloneness. Complete aloneness is an illusion, the opposition between individuality and collectivity a false opposition, fear of aloneness a false fear. The fear of silence is more a fear of its concomitant solitude, the fear of individuality a fear of the void, the centrifugal movement a flight from that which exists not.

Therapy and normalisation

We create that which we fear and fear that which exists not. We therefore create nothingness, a void, hence the phenomenon of the bauble, the emptiness and brittleness inherent in our structures.

Care, cure and therapy, as part and parcel of the medical model, fostering dependency, are commonly placed in opposition to normalisation. But normalisation is institutionalisation in a different form. Our flight from the institution has failed to leave behind those elements in it that we most fear: captivity and loss of identity. The staff–client power balance remains unequal, the criteria of normality are defined by the system, and society itself becomes the institution, with ego-materialistic projectionism its ruling force. There is an ironic reversal: the movement from therapy to normalisation takes us in the opposite direction to that which we think. Therapy is seen as interventionist, a process to which the client is subjected. To the ancient Greeks, *therapia* meant cure but it also meant waiting on or standing beside. Cure or care were much closer to the idea of attention and being than they are in the modern West. Healing had more in common with Simone Weil's notion of waiting than with active, imposed treatment. Therapy is similar in meaning to counselling – sitting down with. It should have the opposite meaning to that with which it has been attributed, whereas normalisation usurps a place for which it is ill fitted. Normalisation fails to do that for which it is designed, to dispense with categories of sick and well, normal and abnormal, whereas *therapia* transcends these boundaries, not confining itself to the realms of 'dis-ease'. It is an essential part of our humanity, being concerned with attention and the primary element, relationship, albeit entwined with the mystery of suffering. Cure is another word for care and care is not intervention but love, attention. Normalisation is concerned with the external; *therapia* with the internal. The centrality of relationship incorporates the centrality of suffering, which is emphasised by both Jungian psychology and Christianity. Art therapy, because it introduces creation, produces the reflective trinity of relationship, suffering and creation, and cannot be other than a spiritual and holistic process.

Resolution

Eastern cultures perceive existence as circular, whereas Western thought is linear. Linearity arises from the dichotomy between internal and external which, like individuality and relationship, we mistakenly perceive as being in opposition. Where a word ends in '-ity' or '-ism', '-ity' denotes natural occurrence, '-ism' deliberate imposition; for example, objectivity – objectivism, activity – activism, duality – dualism. Our false oppositions are dualisms, unnatural divisions, rather than dualities, complementary partnerships. Circular thinking apprehends infinity, linear thinking is finite, hence the proliferation of plurals: skills, goals, aims, objectives. Hierarchy is compatible with linear but not with circular images, which is why the element of domination lingers in normalisation. The disjunction between internal and external arises from the attempt to create closed categories, to separate finite from infinite. The French philosopher, Pascal (1955) writes: 'Le finit s'aneantit en presence de l'infini et deviant un pur neant.' Finite is illusory, therefore, by taking into account the finite alone, we create a void.

In the opening sentences of this chapter, I seemed to take the opposite view to that which followed by suggesting that the deliberate exclusion, in counselling, of elements foreign to attention, could be destructive. That which is sought too hard is inevitably lost. Obsessive focusing on the centre, to the exclusion of the external, involves splitting. You cease to give true attention and begin to play a role. The opposite, emphasising the external without reference to the internal, equally results in impoverishment and fragmentation. The former entails self-destruction; the latter hollowness and implosion. The admittance of foreign elements – for example, advice in counselling or technical help in art therapy, provided these do not take over – connects inner and outer worlds.

I seem to argue against myself but what I am advocating is not substitution of external for internal but reconciliation, a redressing of the balance, a filling in of the centre to give the external greater meaning. This can occur both intra-psychically and organisationally. It is a 'both . . . and' not an 'either . . . or' situation. Goals become valid only if rooted in purpose.

One person in the survey spoke of 'challenge and resting simultaneously', which touched on a vital point. We presuppose opposition between active and passive. Rest is the antithesis of activity, leisure is the antithesis of work. By separating activity from its ground, attention, we create a dualism between active and passive. Activity becomes activism. We start with external instead of internal, thus perpetuating linear thinking and hierarchy. But Pascal saw active and passive not merely as a duality, with activity proceeding out of attentive stillness, but as a unity. To describe this, he used the word 'repos', literally translated as 'rest' but meaning, in Pascal's thought, an active stillness or passive action, a single act of contemplation pervading the whole of life. The reconnections once having been made between East and West, intuition and reason, individuality and collectivity, we regain not only dualities, as opposed to dualisms, but also unities. And we discover further the truth of duality and unity as a unity in themselves, the unity in diversity that touches on the mystery of trinity, this being the idea of two modes unified by a third element. The centrality of suffering also incorporates the ideas of death and life, grief and joy, tragedy and comedy as not merely opposite sides of a coin but as two ends meeting, giving a circular rather than a linear image, a single reality.

I have made extensive use of imagery and semantics for the evocation of ideas and have written from a very personal standpoint. I close with a poem of my own that attempts to express the unity of opposites, the taking up of negative into positive, though without its annihilation, and the sense of the transcendent which projectionist thinking too effectively denies.

Transfiguration
Anger on the surface like a forest fire burning,
Anger deeply buried,
Like crystals,
Cold, impacted, calcified,
But crystals can be made into jewels.

In the bright darkness,
Where silence is music
And stillness dancing,
The foundry thunders,
The unceasing anvils
Hammer out their precious wares,
Suffering, the stuff of Glory,
Pain, the clay of priceless settings,
No journey to be made,
Only a waiting
On the silence music,
And stillness dancing.
The tragi-comic mask revolves,
Whirls, spins,
Ever faster,
Merging,
Not two but one.
All, in the end, is laughter.

References

Freud S (1933/1964) New introductory lectures in psychoanalysis. New York: Norton.
Pascal (1955) Pensées. Paris: Textes de l'Edition Brunschvicg (Garnier).
Weil S (1973) Waiting on God. London: Fontana.

Index